Nurses, Jobs and Resumes

Resume Revisions for RNs
From the New Grad RN to the Experienced RN

Cover-art-photography:
Capture the Canvas Photography: Mikayla Kosicek

Cover graphic designer: Joyce Fler-Reyes

Interior graphic designer: Abul Ala Muhammad Iqbal

Editor: Author Bridge Media, Formerly Ocean Cloud Media: Helen Chang

Publishing Company: Visionary LLC

Proudly Printed in the United States of America

First paperback printing: November 2014

ISBN-10: 0985755202
ISBN-13: 978-0-9857552-0-1

Published Books

Nurses, Jobs and Money
A Guide to Advancing Your Nursing Career and Salary

Nurses, Jobs and Resumes
Resume Revisions for RNs From the New Grad RN to the Experienced RN

Coming Soon:

Nurses, Jobs and Education

Foreign Educated RNs Coming to America

CONTENTS

DEDICATION

To my parents, for having the courage to change their environment, which in turn afforded me a more educated and open-minded environment to grow up and thrive in.

To my father-in-law and mother-in-law, for raising a wonderful son who has become an inspirational husband and father.

To my husband and children, for making everything possible, cheering me on when I am discouraged, putting up with my high energy, and making me laugh and notice the little things in life.

And to the numerous nurses, new grad RNs, and experienced RNs, who have put aside traditional ideas, trusted in me, and are now soaring to new heights in their nursing careers!

ACKNOWLEDGMENTS

The continued belief in what I do and positive attitude of the nurses who work with me is what keeps me going after what I firmly believe I'm meant to do: help nurses realize the multifaceted opportunities that are open to them in nursing, and what they are truly able to do with the degree in nursing that they already have.

My husband Mike, although he is not a nurse, has learned a great deal about nursing employment possibilities. He is particularly strategic in helping nurses see the bigger vision of what they can do with the degree and background they already have. When the nurses he speaks with opt to work with me as a mentor, I lead them step-by-step to make their love of nursing flourish again and help them to once more be happy in their work.

Thank you, Mike, for all of your help and sharing in the excitement of helping nurses fall in love with nursing all over again, and for taking their initial calls, and explaining how I can help.

Our son Blake continues to be instrumental in his ongoing assistance with my techie issues. His kindness, patience, and keen insights are invaluable, as is his hands-on learning style for the Apple products we exclusively use. Although my learning is slow at times, I deeply thank him and appreciate his insights and teaching style.

In case you do not realize how funny that is, we homeschool our children. Blake is clearly not taking techie insights from his teachers, but rather, he is a self-taught, thanks to YouTube. Blake is the home computer guy, who in turn has kindly taught his teachers the techie updates.

Our daughter, and Capture the Canvas Photography (found on Facebook) owner, Mikaya Kosicek, is the creative magic behind the nursing pictures on my website, Facebook page, and books. I am not a fan of "normal" photos and Mikayla has added fun into the shots with the nurses, which exemplifies the fun that this wonderful profession can hold.

Thank you, Mikayla, for capturing those moments—and many more—in such an innovative way!

The team at Author Bridge Media, formerly Ocean Cloud Media Inc., was so wonderful to work with on my first book, *Nurses, Jobs and Money — A Guide To Advancing Your Nursing Career and Salary*, that there was no doubt in my mind when it came to having them join my team again. The numerous nurses who have worked with me over the years told me they could hear me as they read through the pages of my book. That is true talent —pure talent for a journalist, and I applaud Helen Chang and her team.

I have such great respect and dedication for my internal graphic designer, Abul Ala Muhammad Iqbal. Iqbal's hard work and dedication to my projects make them as special as if he was working on his own manuscript. He paid attention to detail on everything and made sure I was pleased with his finishing touches on my work.

My cover graphic designer, Joyce Fler-Reyes, continues to be professional and honest as to what appears best visually for consumers, as she shares multiple examples and her invaluable insights.

Thank you to the nurses who reached out to me on Facebook at my Nursing Career Professionals page when I posted an open casting call for "before" resumes. These nurses openly and willingly sent me their "before" resumes for use in this book for everyone to learn from. As a given, I've changed the names and other personalized information on the resumes showcased in this book, but the rest of the information is real.

One by one, in fair trade, I spent time on the phone with the nurses who openly shared the "before" resumes, that you will see in this book. For those who volunteered in this way, I helped them learn how to best showcase themselves to take advantage of the endless opportunities that are open to them in their marketplaces using the degree that they already have.

I had so much fun helping these nurses, each and every one of them! I thank them all for allowing other nurses to learn from their mistakes so that we can advance as a profession by learning from one another.

As in so many aspects of life, it takes a village, and in writing a book, that is no different. Without my village, my books' success would not be what it is today, making a positive impact on the multiple generations of nurses who reach out to read innovative and cutting edge insights from a nurse who understands the changing environment of healthcare, and what it takes to positively position nurses ahead of that curve.

Introduction

Nurses should love what they are doing, be it in traditional bedside nursing employment venues or beyond.

Most new grads and experienced nurses alike are unaware of all of the amazing employment opportunities they have within nursing.

True, you may have heard that there are endless possibilities as a nurse. But other than listing off those job titles, it's likely that no one has ever shown you how to find those jobs, let alone what you need to put on your resume to get noticed for them.

I'm willing to bet that this is because the people you have listened to in the past have only worked in traditional nursing employment venues.

Well, all that is about to change. I've worked in traditional and nontraditional nursing employment venues, and I can show you what it takes to work in both of those environments!

True, as an RN, you could work in traditional nursing employment venues such as a hospital, doctor's office, clinic or traditional education. However, you may also choose a different path in nursing. You have what it takes to land a job in a nontraditional employment venue—even as a new grad!

Nurses are needed in both the traditional and nontraditional nursing employment arenas. Both new grad nurses *and* experienced nurses can positively impact healthcare and patients in these nursing employment venues by using their critical thinking and nursing skillsets.

But what are these nontraditional nursing employment venues, and how do you know if they would be of interest to you? Let's take a closer look at this.

A World of Possibilities

First off, no job title is as important as the characteristics that the position entails. For example, do you prefer to go to a single location and stay there for eight or more hours, or do you prefer to be more mobile as you work?

Do you prefer to have the same coworkers day in and day out, or do you like to interact with different people? Day shift, afternoon, or nights? Call? No call? Weekends, or no weekends? These are just a few of the possibilities available when you look at the numerous employment options in nursing.

You can start by simply looking at titles, to see if any of these intrigue you. Have you considered positions as a field nurse case manager, or perhaps a telephonic nurse case manager? Or maybe infusion nursing, dialysis nursing, or even home health nursing may be more to your liking.

Do you like computers? If so, have you ever thought about a nursing informatics role, or being a nurse in EMR implementation?

Are you outgoing? Then what about a job in sales or sales support as a nurse, nurse educator, or medical science liaison?

How about risk management, utilization review, occupational health, hospice, or wellness nursing?

There are so many opportunities open to you as a nurse, from the newly graduated to the experienced RN—with a diploma, associate's, bachelor's, master's, and beyond!

While many falsely assume that more education will help you to land a position, the real truth is that a great resume is the key first step to getting the job you really want in nursing.

Being open-minded and realizing what qualifications really are or are not needed and appropriately showcasing your current skillset on the resume is the key to getting the conversation that leads to a job offer.

Until now, you have most likely been blocking the window of opportunity to these conversations due to the outdated information on your resume.

Why do I say that?

I say it because I've personally experienced this in my nursing career and in the nursing careers of those I've helped. I've seen both new grads and experienced nurses with outdated techniques used on their resumes. And you know what? Their phone never, or rarely, rings with opportunities.

More often than not, nurses have not learned what they truly can do outside of traditional nursing employment venues. Likewise, they're often unaware of the required language and preferred meanings associated with these kinds of opportunities.

As a result of this lack of knowledge, it's common for these nurses to unintentionally and unnecessarily sabotage their own chances when applying for these kinds of jobs.

So what makes me uniquely qualified to help you?

I have a multifaceted background in nursing, ranging from traditional nursing employment in bedside nursing, hospital nursing unit director, correctional nursing, hospice, community health nursing, collegiate nursing professor and management to nontraditional nursing employment in pharmaceutical sales, clinical nurse educator in biotech, and more.

What's more, I am an instrumental leader who has been able to assist other nurses (both new grads and experienced RNs) replicate my success in their own careers and in their own markets across this great nation—in both traditional and nontraditional employment venues for nursing.

We're talking about learning from someone who has been where you want to be, versus learning from someone who has not done what you want to do. It's a night and day difference.

Knowing firsthand about the ins and outs, network access, and other useful details included in this book will enhance your success—both in your nursing career journey and when it comes landing the position that you desire, or even by simply pointing you in a more desirable direction if you do not currently know the full array of options available to you.

Are you ready to have your phone ring and to discuss the wide range of amazing opportunities in nursing that are available to you?

Are you ready to have your working conditions, hours, and workdays geared to your lifestyle?

Are you excited about making more income while doing something that you love, without necessarily going for more college degrees first?

Are you thrilled at the possibility of impacting healthcare on a small or large level?

Does your heart race with excitement when you realize that you can blend what you like to do outside of work with your work in nursing?

If you answered yes to any of these questions, then you'll need to apply for these jobs using a big bucks resume that gets you noticed. You cannot begin to have these discussions if your resume is less than great, and if it is not making your phone ring.

My next question is would you like to be the one with multiple offers for amazing positions in nursing?

If so, do you have a big bucks resume?

No?

Well, there is no need to panic if you don't yet have this amazing tool in your job-seeking arsenal. Most nurses do not have a big bucks resume. This is great news, because as you learn how to create a big bucks resume, you will stand out above your competition!

The biggest problem with an outdated resume chock full of outdated techniques is that it limits the extended opportunities for employment and nursing career growth.

New grads and experienced nurses from across the country seem to have a common problem with this. They're using resumes filled with outdated techniques, combined with a lack of appropriately showcasing their true skillset using the solid rationales and proof of their impact.

It's these missing or inadequate pieces that will cause a potential employer to skip over an otherwise well-qualified nurse's resume in favor of someone who knows how to do this well.

Most nurses do not realize that a big bucks resume will not only make their phone ring, but will aid in the interview too!

A big bucks resume is not only a tool for the nurse to use to apply for jobs, but it will make recruiters for amazing jobs actually seek out that nurse for the jobs they're trying to fill.

So, what is needed to put together a big bucks resume?

- A big bucks resume is a working document that needs to be personalized to each and every person.
- A big bucks resume needs to showcase previous work experience in a manner that directly relates to the job the applicant is presently seeking.
- A big bucks resume will showcase the infusion of the business in healthcare into the practice of healthcare, as well as one's impactful results in that business.

The time has arrived for you to learn how to make your resume a big bucks resume. And you'll be learning this from a nurse who has firsthand experience across traditional and nontraditional employment venues, not only in nursing, but as a nurse who has helped thousands of other nurses bridge this gap. And now it is your turn.

Your new big bucks resume will open endless doors of opportunities and avenues for you to expand your nursing career!

Chapter 1:Navigating the Nursing Job-Search Landscape

Get the Lay of the Land

Marketing makes the world go around!

Have you noticed all of the social media marketing from companies such as Facebook? Yes, it is a bit creepy that whatever you search for online at big-box stores then shows up on your Facebook social media ads, emulating your latest search!

Have you noticed this?

Although it can seem a little creepy, it is actually pure genius.

Are you being genius in your marketing? When you search for a new position, you are marketing yourself.

How are you marketing yourself?

If you have been using the 'spray and pray' method with your outdated resume, you are tainting and massively contaminating your marketplace. And you are in for a wake-up call.

To be clear, the spray and pray method is when you apply for any position that has RN in the title, all over your local area, where you are seeking employment. When you do this, you are not being strategic in what you are applying for. Instead, you are spraying your information out there to all of those places.

Stop the spray and pray today!

Why? Is it really that bad of a marketing maneuver?

Think about it.

You apply online nowadays. If you put your information into the computer and you are not showcasing yourself strategically, when you reapply to the same employer six, twelve, eighteen, or twenty-four months down the road, the computer recognizes it is you again. You did not meet the qualifications previously, so why would they want you now?!

If you want a particular type of position, you need to strategically apply and track how long it takes to hear from the employer.

If you are not time-tracking after applying, and you keep applying and applying in your marketplace, you are diminishing your chances of gainful employment. Sadly, in this case, your timeframe for finding gainful employment could span a few years.

In other words, stop tainting and contaminating your marketplace right now or you will have to move away to get work!

The good news is that this can be avoided. In this book, I'm going to teach you how to be strategic in your approach to your job hunt so that you can actually land the job you really want and advance your career in nursing.

I've found that most nursing schools do not show nurses what they really can do as a nurse other than traditional employment venue roles.

This does not surprise me, as many of the nursing faculty themselves have never done anything other than traditional nursing. True, they are very seasoned nurses, but often they have only had positions as a nurse within traditional employment venues.

The bottom line is that people tend to teach what they know and have experienced.

I am here to say that it is time for a different teacher, a different nurse, a different voice to be heard for the RNs.

In this chapter, I'll teach you how to recognize and perfectly position yourself to seize the endless opportunities available to you in the field of nursing, including a breakdown of nontraditional nursing roles and the business of nursing.

Employment Venues for Nurses

Nontraditional Employment Venues for Nurses

Not sure yet what nontraditional employment venues for nurses are?

When I say nontraditional employment venues for nurses, I'm talking about nurses in dialysis, hospice, case management, informatics, navigators, liaisons, wellness, worker's compensation, occupational health, educators, marketing, administrators, sales, utilization review, documentation, correctional, specialists, and more.

I've outlined in depth how to search for nontraditional and traditional nursing jobs in my first book, *Nurses, Jobs and Money — A Guide to Advancing Your Nursing Career and Salary.*

The key now is learning how to create a big bucks resume that will get you noticed for these jobs!

Traditional Employment Venues for Nurses

So what do I mean by traditional roles? Namely, I mean being a nurse in a hospital, doctor's office or clinic.

Advanced practice and traditional collegiate teaching roles are also traditional roles or traditional employment venues for nurses.

Most nurses make lateral moves, from one hospital department to another, and so on. I often find that if nurses go for more higher education, most then go on to teach nursing or become advanced practice nurses.

There is nothing wrong with these traditional roles for those that want them, but there are others out there who want more.

The cycle in nursing that pushes most nurses towards traditional employment venues for nurses continues, in my opinion, because those who go on to teach are the ones who have mainly only been in those same traditional nursing employment roles. So of course, these are the roles they tell new RNs about, and they give only very limited information on other facets of nursing let alone the valuable insights on how to get into the other facets of nursing.

They mainly speak of what they already know from their own limited experience.

I feel it is time for this cycle to be broken.

It is time to truly teach RNs what they really can do within the profession of nursing, using the degree they already have.

Please understand, I am not against seeking further education. But sadly, I hear from too many RNs across this nation who are returning for higher and higher degrees in nursing, and still find themselves out of work. Unfortunately, by then, they are strapped with massive student loan debt.

There is a different way.

I know how to teach and lead RNs who aspire to do more in their career because I've done it myself, and I've helped other nurses to go on and have a multifaceted career in nursing as well.

I know how to positively position nursing students for a

career in nursing, not merely a job.

Because I see a much bigger picture of real possibilities in nursing, I am able to help strategically position nurses of all experience levels for a bright career in nursing focused on their personal strengths and desires.

The Disconnect

Unfortunately, I've found that many of the higher-ups in nursing education do not embrace the necessary changes that are needed to help future nursing professionals reach both traditional and nontraditional nursing employment venues.

I have even heard from two huge nursing book publishing companies that there is not a need for the information that I am sharing.

Sad, because I know this need exists.

Colleges are starting to realize this need now that the second largest for-profit system folded due in part to its new grads not landing jobs in their field of study. This was the fate of Corinthian Colleges, Inc., whose nursing college was under the name Everest. A quick Google search will give you a fuller picture of this story if you want to know more.

I have been told by top nursing leaders that there is not an employment challenge out there for new grads or older, seasoned RNs. I shake my head and refuse to listen to this, because through my interactions with people across this nation, I know better.

Another quick Google search of unemployed RNs, from the newly graduated to experienced RNs, will demonstrate this need. The stories of the RNs in groups on LinkedIn.com alone reveal the sad realities of nursing unemployment, told by those who are not able to find positions as new grad RNs and even experienced RNs.

Part of this is because experienced nurses who have been away from the bedside for two years or longer are now being looked at as new grad RNs. These well-seasoned RNs are even more challenged when it comes to landing job interviews because they are seen as brand new and, quite frankly, they command a higher wage due to their longer experience.

This is not a good fit for a hospital system that is challenged with cost containment and the need for slimming and trimming budgets.

Monthly Earning Losses

I know the statistics.

Everything I'm telling you is here for a reason and backed up by reliable sources.

For example, a retrospective analysis published in 2014 showed that in 2013, 43 percent of newly graduated RNs were unable to find gainful employment in nursing for six to eighteen months after graduation.

Often, these newly graduated RNs leave the field of nursing because they need income to repay their student loans. This saddens me greatly, even as it fuels me to continue my journey to showcase a different way to build a career in nursing using my own innovative insights to change these unfortunate statistics.

The cost of unemployment is high. Very high.

Think about that.

The national average hourly pay for a RN is $25 per hour. That comes out to about $52,000 a year.

So for every month that passes while a newly graduated RN is unemployed, he or she is losing more than $4,300 of income.

Why are you choosing to lose over $4,300 a month? You may say that you are not choosing that path, but you are if you continue to do what you are presently doing without changing anything and are expecting a different result.

If you have not had offers that led to a solid position, whatever it is that you are doing is clearly not working. Period.

To be fully transparent, by not changing what you are doing, it is your choice to lose money. So yes, you are choosing to lose over $4,300 a month.

Stop it.

There is something different that you can do!

You are in the right spot to learn what you can do to positively position yourself in your marketplace.

The National Perspective

With the position that I am in, I hear from RNs from across the nation, new grad and experienced RNs alike, who cannot find jobs in nursing.

Stop listening to the colleges who say what a wonderful job market there is for nurses. That is true for experienced nurses who are under fifty and still at the bedside. Really.

Another quick Google search will show you what is happening to the older experienced nurses: age discrimination, difficulty landing jobs, or a huge cut in pay required to find gainful employment in nursing.

If a nurse has stepped away from the bedside for two years or more, even those positions are out of reach!

So is there hope?

Yes! And with my expertise in and expanded vision of our profession, I can offer you that hope.

I have strategic and national proven step-by-step techniques that help RNs across the experience and age spectrum to not only find jobs in nursing, but to land them!

I have a much bigger view of the problems in the employment venues for nursing than just the small view from a local school, college, or university.

Additionally, I have the advantage of a blended view of nursing and business. This is key, because healthcare really is a business, and it is a big business. The same goes for nursing education—it is also a big business.

It pains me that this is happening and that no one is teaching a different way forward for nurses, perhaps because they don't know or they are not open to change, or perhaps because the people up top made the decision that this information was not needed.

For whatever reason it is happening, the result is that this important information never made it to those who fell into the 43 percent of newly graduated RNs who were unable to find gainful employment in nursing for six to eighteen months after graduation.

These newly graduated RNs, who have spent thousands and thousands of dollars to earn their degree, come to me in a panic, because they know that the next wave of new grad RNs will be graduating merely one semester, or quarter, from now.

And that if they don't act soon, they will be swept out to sea as the next wave of new grads crashes in on their market, yet again flooding the area with new RN grads.

I also hear from experienced RNs who are in a panic because they have never been unemployed before and now cannot land a job in nursing.

The traditional nursing employers are not willing to pay top dollar anymore nor risk injury with older RNs. Instead, they can get an RN with a few years of experience under his or her belt for a fraction of the price, not to mention have a younger worker who stereotypically may have more energy and less health issues. I know—*stereotypically* speaking is the key word there.

Wake up, nurses.

This has been happening across various industries.

Why would you falsely believe this would not happen in healthcare and in nursing?

It is.

Yet many won't speak of this obvious truth.

I will.

Nursing has changed. So has our economy.

I feel it is better to understand what is going on in the marketplace so you can strategically position yourself ahead of the curve and be desirable to potential employers.

I will teach you how to overcome this, and how to positively position yourself to be noticed, starting with your resume. In this book, you'll learn how to utilize a current resume to get interviews and, ultimately, to land the job!

I'm about to teach you how to carry a personal safety net wherever you go, all the time!

This personal employment safety net is strategic and innovative, and it has been proven to work across the nation.

Yes, it will take time to learn, but once fully grasped, you will have this knowledge with you forever. Arm in arm, I will walk you though this process, so that you learn and understand the key points and rationale before I release you into the marketplace.

If it sounds like I'm reading your mind, I agree—this should be a fundamental learning building block in college prior to graduation. Again, I'm working on that too. Times have changed and so too should our nursing courses!

Be Strategic

There is a strategic plan that I initially implemented with new grad RNs and have expanded to be used by experienced RNs as well.

This plan has proven—time and time again, no matter how massively a particular market is flooded—how to positively penetrate the market to find work and gain much-needed experience.

I know how to build the base of experience wide and

quickly for the newly graduated. More often then not, this in turn then aids the new grad RN to land the position that he or she was initially seeking.

Again, I fully outlined this in my first book, *Nurses, Jobs and Money — A Guide To Advancing Your Nursing Career and Salary*. If you have not already, pick up a copy so that you understand what, how, and why to do things strategically to win!

The solutions I present work not only for newly graduated RNs, but experienced RNs too. With the right strategy, the hiring stumbling blocks of age discrimination and higher hourly wage earnings can be overcome.

The Resume

Although there are many steps in my strategic plan to gainful nursing employment, the resume is the center focus for most of these.

Countless nurses from across the nation have reached out to me. What many of them falsely believe is that they only need help with creating a big bucks resume.

Again, I firmly believe that a resume is only one facet of the overall employment picture. For example, job searching, the game of online applications, interviewing, salary negotiations, and more all play a vital role for RNs in landing the job they are seeking.

However, as I have helped RNs across the country, I keep running into train wreck resumes. And I realized the need to address this particular facet on its own.

Outdated Techniques

First of all, the information you were taught to put on your resume in college or from nursing colleagues is more than likely outdated.

Why would I go out on a limb and say such a thing?

Because I've seen it time and time again. This issue crops up constantly in my work with new grads and experienced nurses.

Every day I see nurses who are implementing the outdated techniques that their schools, colleges, universities, and nursing colleagues are continuing to tell them to use. These nurses then scratch their heads in wonder as to why they are not landing interviews and then jobs.

But I have a current perspective. And I have a question that I really want you to think about . . .

A Current Perspective

Be honest.

Look at the person or people who are giving you your advice on resumes, interviews, and the like. When was the last time he or she had to look for a job in this economy? More likely then not, it was more than one year, five years or even fifteen years ago.

Nursing today is not the same as your mother's nursing.

Nursing today is often for those that are the breadwinners for their family.

Nursing today is different. And yes, I see things differently.

As healthcare is changing in this nation, so too must the resumes of healthcare workers!

To prove that what I say is true, I will show you examples from across the nation that contain specific instances of the outdated techniques I'm talking about. From there, I will explain how to overcome these outdated techniques and explain the rationale as to why I do things differently and how this will help you.

What I will not do is give you a cookie-cutter format for a resume.

Why?

No matter who writes it for you, a cookie-cutter resume will not help you get to where you want to be in your nursing career.

Make It Great

A big bucks resume needs to be personalized.

A big bucks resume is a working document for you to use to strategically position yourself above the competition, and to get an interview that leads to a job offer.

The one hundred and one interview questions method does not work. In your interview, you need to work off of your big bucks resume with relevant examples of what you did and the impact you made doing it.

A big bucks resume is a working document that needs to be personalized to each and every person.

A big bucks resume needs to showcase previous work experience in a manner that directly relates to the job the applicant is presently seeking.

A big bucks resume is not a one-size-fits-all. That is why I vehemently refuse to post a ton of "after" examples of resumes, because otherwise, you will continue to get the same results you are currently getting rather than the results you are dreaming of.

A big bucks resume is simply not something that you can download from the internet, nor something you can pay to have written for you by someone who never speaks with you and doesn't understand how to blend nursing and the business of healthcare.

Rather, a big bucks resume is personalized by someone who has insights about how to help you get to where you want to go in nursing—because they understand what it takes to get you there.

So if you genuinely want to learn how to write a big bucks resume that will make you stand out, be noticed, and be memorable, while highlighting the skillset you truly offer an employer and showcasing the infusion of the business in healthcare, get ready!

Get Ready to Be Great

If you want a big bucks resume that will land you a job, either in traditional or nontraditional nursing employment venues, as a new grad RN or an experienced RN, then jump in!

Go and grab a copy of your resume right now, as you will want to make notes as we move along through my innovative insights.

Together, we will address head on the outdated techniques that new grad RNs and experienced RNs are using on resumes. I'll explain why that outdated verbiage is not working for RNs to help them strategically land jobs.

The Business of Healthcare

What is the business of healthcare?

As soon as I start to describe this, you will realize you already know what I'm talking about. The trick is being able to convey that you know this to prospective employers.

Think about it. Whether a business is for-profit or not-for-profit, the goal of any business is to make money.

The same is true in healthcare.

As a nurse, you are asked to do more and more and to spend less and less, or to do more with less and less—from supplies to staff.

Sounds familiar, right?

That is cost containment. Yes, that is a business term!

What about decreasing budgets by lowering the amount of overtime?

Again, that's business.

Customer service?

Yes, business-related.

Healthcare *is* a business. The corporations that often own the doctor's office, the hospital, and even the collegiate institutions are *business*-minded. Healthcare is too.

The biggest disconnect is with healthcare providers, as many have never looked at what they truly are doing. They are doing business—specifically, the business of healthcare.

Think about it as a nurse. Here is a scenario to ponder. Let's say you see "X" amount more patients per day than your coworker.

If a patient visit earns the business $100.00, and you see five more patients per week than your coworkers, then you have easily generated $500.00+ more income per week for your employer.

Now extrapolate that out for the entire year. That is over $25,000 of extra income you are making for your employer, be it a doctor's office, hospital, or some other venue.

Interestingly, if you are like the nurse in our example, you most likely make the same amount of money as your coworker—even if you do more work!

We have all been in work environments where one coworker outperforms another. Perhaps in the past you have worked in fast food, the bank, or at the mall, and you have seen this same scenario play out there.

The point is, if you consistently get more work done than your coworkers, you need to showcase this on your healthcare resume as a nurse, so you can start to be paid what you are worth!

But is this possible for the new grad? Yes!

New grads fall into the trap of using the same outdated techniques, failing to incorporate the business of healthcare, listing off tasks instead of showcasing results, and more on their resumes.

Worse yet, new grads are making the outdated and yet hallmark mistake of actually listing their mandated clinical rotations on their resume! This outdated advice continues to be taught from generation to generation in nursing schools. It is time for a different approach for our profession, because this outdated technique is no longer working.

New grad RNs, there is an entire chapter in this book that will give you resume examples, along with insights and in-depth explanations about why you should not put your clinical rotations on your resume. The truth is that this negatively affects you!

I know, I know—your college is actually encouraging you to list your clinicals, but I will specifically challenge you with solid and sound rationales for today's job market on why this is a big mistake.

In the next chapter, I will explain not only how to make your resume current, but to make it stand out above the competition. You will learn what needs to be on your resume to make your phone ring with opportunities, and how to create your own safety net that will follow you wherever you go, all of the time!

Additionally, if you would like to see and hear me talk about resume do's and don'ts, you can watch my free video series at http://carmenk.crystalcleardm.com/.

Chapter 2: Dispelling the Myths of the Nursing Job Hunt

If *The Tonight Show* host Jimmy Fallon focused on having guests on the show from twenty or more years ago, I guarantee you it would not be the highest rated evening show.

Staying current, be it in American pop culture, music, or resumes, is huge. Being current drives attention. Being current creates interest. Being current leads to opportunities.

Experienced nurses and newly graduated nurses from both regionally and nationally accredited programs of all levels (ADN, BSN, and even MSN and beyond) are all using outdated techniques on their resumes. They are not staying current in what employers are seeking: the blending of nursing and business.

Staying Current

The bigger question then, is *why* are nurses not staying current with respect to their resumes?

Often, it is because those they are learning from those who have not looked for a job in nursing in a long, long time.

Additionally, it is often that those they are learning from have only worked in the traditional roles of nursing.

Again, there is nothing wrong with choosing a traditional path in nursing. But if you are seeking something different in your own nursing career, you need to learn a different way forward.

And even though you may have been in your current nursing role for a long time, you are not necessarily safe. No job is safe. Downsizing does and will happen.

Healthcare is changing, and so too should your resume.

In this chapter, I will teach you how to stay current, get noticed, and open countless doors of opportunities in nursing!

I will teach you how to showcase your true skillset—the skillset that numerous employers highly desire—so that if and when you are downsized, you will feel confident in your ability to secure gainful employment in another facet of nursing.

Changes

Even if you want to stay in traditional nursing, you need to be cognizant of the fact that healthcare itself is changing.

The hospital, doctor's office, clinic, or educational system in your area is more than likely now a part of a bigger system.

Corporations are now controlling community hospitals and even collegiate systems.

The nursing positions of the past were pretty straightforward and, overall, most RNs have not changed how they present themselves on paper in a resume as the years have gone by. But times have changed.

Healthcare has changed.

The chances of you being downsized as a nurse in traditional or nontraditional employment venues are huge!

Rather than being a sitting duck, I will teach you how to be current. The techniques that I will teach you will afford you a personal safety net to use for wherever and whenever you go!

Education

Let me make this very clear: you can do a lot with the degree you already have in nontraditional employment venues for nursing.

The traditional employment venues for nursing will ask for more and more experience, and will require more and more pieces of paper, and yet you will work for less and less pay, and not have as many benefits as you will in nontraditional nursing employment venues.

Many people keep returning to school for more and more pieces of paper, falsely believing this is the only way to advance their nursing careers. It is not.

With first hand experience, I am here to tell you that even with my Certificate in Nurse-Midwifery and a 4.0 GPA in grad school from Case Western Reserve University with my MSN, I only needed my MSN for four of the jobs I've ever had.

Which ones did I need a master's degree for?

A masters degree was required for my positions teaching in collegiate nursing, working as an APRN, for the Director of Nursing position at Corinthian College, and as the Associate Dean of Nursing in a collegiate setting.

No, I did not need my MSN to be the unit director of women's health, nor to be a staff nurse, pharmaceutical sales representative, nurse educator, author, or speaker.

Interestingly, I was happier in other roles, such as a clinical nurse educator for inVentiv Health with Johnson & Johnson as an example. At this job and others like it, I earned more and had more time freedom than I did in my other positions. Just for the record, although preferred, you do not have to have a bachelor's degree for the position that I've enjoyed the most!

Knowing how to showcase your experience appropriately will often trump your degrees when you seek employment in nontraditional employment venues for nursing.

Literally, companies are simply waiting for nurses with great experience highlighted appropriately on their resumes to apply!

Same Role

If you have been in the same position for twenty or more years, you still can make a move to something else!

True, the learning curve of any new job just stinks. Think about it. You cannot even answer the phone right when you start at a new position, because inevitably someone will have the wrong extension and ask you to transfer them, and you have no idea where to transfer them to!

Starting new at anything—really, change of any kind—can be nerve-wracking.

Is it worth it?

Absolutely!

Why?

Think of it from the employer's standpoint. Would you rather hire someone who had experience at one place, or varied experiences to draw upon?

Or look at it this way. If you needed brain surgery, would you want a surgeon who has been at a variety of hospitals, seen many cases, learned different ways of dealing with his or her OR team, is up on various techniques, and is current with all kinds of technology?

Or would you want a surgeon who has been at one place, who has seen a lot of things, but has done everything the same way?

I'd want someone who had the various experiences and insights. The fresher ideas, different ways of looking at a similar issue, experiences interacting with different people, exemplifying how you can get along with others, and familiarity with different technologies is what I'd prefer. And so would many employers.

More than likely, you will not retire from where you are currently employed, even if you have been there for twenty years. I say that with confidence because of what is happening in our economy across other industries. People a few months or a few years from retirement are suddenly getting downsized.

Since that is how things are now, why would you wait and not broaden your experience?

Fear?

Not an option.

Traditional employment venues in nursing no longer make you safe by default as a nurse anymore. Nurses a few years away from retirement in traditional employment venues across the country are being downsized.

With the techniques I'm about to teach you, you will not only carry a personal safety net wherever you go, you will gain the business insights as to how your daily actions directly impact the corporate outcomes!

I'll teach you how to showcase your experience so you are solid, strong, and able to advance your career so that you are better able to care for yourself and your family.

Hopelessly Doomed

If you feel that you cannot do anything different because of your degree or past experience, take a deep breath. I've already addressed this false claim. You absolutely can do something different.

What if you don't feel you can do anything different due to your location or disability?

You are no longer hopelessly doomed!

Why? Because work-at-home positions are all over the place now.

Having a big bucks resume will once more position you at the head of the pack for amazing opportunities!

New Grad

Believe it or not, you really do not have to work in a hospital on a med-surg floor for one to three years for someone to hire you in nursing.

The patients are no longer in the hospital.

Think about it.

You could have a double mastectomy this morning and the odds are extremely high—even likely—that you would be discharged home tonight!

True, you would still have your drains, and possibly a pain

pump and all, but you would be home because the risk of succumbing to a nosocomial infection at the hospital is greater than the risk of succumbing to surgical complications. Thus, your recovery is more positively favored in your own home.

If the patients are no longer in the hospital as long as they used to be, why are you persisting in the false belief that you must go there to work in order to be a nurse for your first few years? You do not. That is outdated thinking.

There are other opportunities for new grads that will actually welcome you with open arms.

Guess what the key is to getting noticed? Right! A big bucks resume.

Let me show you!

Chapter 3: The Key Elements of a Killer Nursing Resume

Desserts are not only pretty, but they taste great!

Made from scratch desserts taste superior to the slice-and-bake desserts that now flood the market.

But why is that?

You simply cannot have a cookie-cutter, slice-and-bake dessert that tastes as great as one made from scratch. The made-from-scratch dessert has fresh ingredients and skips the plethora of preservatives.

How a dessert comes together is all in the details. Unlike cooking, baking requires precise amounts of the required ingredients.

Recipes for desserts delineate how and when the ingredients should be added, as well as how they should be sifted, folded, mixed, and stirred.

Big bucks resumes are no different.

Cookie-cutter resumes flood the market, but are not as great as a made-from-scratch, truly personalized resume.

A big bucks resume is put together following an ingredient list and a set of precise directions regarding what should be added, when, and how.

Just like desserts, there is a rhyme and a reason behind each and every section of a great resume.

Big Bucks Resume Ingredients

The list of things it takes to make a big bucks resume is not long, but just as in baking, each particular ingredient, no matter how big or how small, is imperative for a successful overall outcome.

What are the ingredients for a successful big bucks resume?

- Format and layout
- Name and initials
- Contact info
- Summary
- Experience
- Education

In this chapter, I will specifically take each one of the ingredients from this list and teach you why it is important. This will allow you to create a homemade, from scratch big bucks resume of your own.

All of the examples we will cover are actual resumes that were sent to me from across the nation. As mentioned earlier, the names and contact information has been changed, but I kept everything else the same so that you can get a flavor of the competition in the marketplace.

Get ready!

It is time to dissect a healthcare resume step-by-step, and ingredient-by-ingredient, to learn what is truly needed to transform a cookie-cutter resume into a big bucks resume.

Lets dive right in!

Format and Layout

Picture a magazine cover in your mind, look one up online, or even go to your local supermarket and look at the magazines in the checkout lines.

What do you notice about the magazine covers you see?

I would bet you notice the name of the magazine, the image on the magazine cover, and the verbiage that is on the left, right, and bottom of the magazine cover layout.

Highly trained marketing professionals have spent a lot of time and money on the layout of the magazine cover for one reason: to sell more magazines.

You need to do the same with your resume.

Mirror the traits that the marketing gurus have put into these magazine covers in your resume.

The fonts on the magazines are eye-catching, yet easy to read. Again, reflect back to your resume. It needs to emulate the magazine cover traits.

Although I recommend one uniform font for the entire resume, the size of the font should vary in different sections of the resume to catch the reader's eye.

Each section of the resume has important information and therefore deserves to be visually separate spatially so that the important information is seen. To be clear, you don't want to have the resume visually run together. If your resume does, you risk having the reader not pay attention to the imperative information in each section—information that is needed to put you towards the top of the candidate list.

You can visually command the attention of the reader with this simple trick: vary your font size and appearance.

Step by step, you will learn how to command and maintain the reader's attention.

Just as your eye noticed the name of the magazine and the article highlights listed on the far right, left, and bottom of the magazine, the same should happen with your resume.

Utilize the same font and sprinkle in bold, underlined, and even italicized versions of that font, along with different font sizes for the lettering on different sections.

Why?

To stand out and be noticed!

I'm sure you hear that all the time: "Your resume needs to stand out and be noticed." No one is talking about the type of paper, nor the color of the paper the resume is on. Instead, to stand out and be noticed, you need to start with the visual appeal of the resume.

So this is the first step of being noticed: the format and layout.

Not sure if this really makes a big difference?

Remember, thousands of dollars from numerous marketing teams are poured into magazine covers. These dollars would not be spent if the format and layout really did not make a difference.

Let that sink in.

Now take a look at the difference for yourself with a nursing resume. Remember, this example is given merely to let you see format and layout differences. Do not start copying the verbiage, as I will address this issue separately later on.

Yes, this is a real resume from one of my clients (with the name and other identifying information removed). This was the "before" resume format and layout.

Again, focus on the format and layout, not what is actually written.

Oh My Goodness, BS, RN
1234 NW Main Street
Anywhere, FL 33333
123-456-7890
OhMyGoodness@gmail.com

SKILLS SUMMARY

Active Florida Registered Nurse licenses with over seven years experience working in the acute care setting, understanding the processes and workflow common in this environment; solid customer service background that includes excellent interpersonal skills and the ability to interact positively as part of a multi-disciplinary team. Possess strong critical thinking and decision making abilities; highly analytical. Competent in managing multiple priorities and meeting deadlines. Excellent written and verbal communications skills. Experience working with various computer applications within the acute care setting as well as the business sector. Comfortable working with the internet and technology. Looking for the opportunity to transition into Clinical Informatics.

QUALIFICATIONS

CUSTOMER SERVICE

Competent in communicating with internal and external customers whether in person or by telephone to establish rapport, provide assistance and recommend solutions. Accustom to responding and resolving customer concerns, providing win-win resolutions in response to client inquiries. Responsible for company-client follow-up and liaison which include timely reviews, proficient multi-tasking and meeting tight deadlines.

INTERPERSONAL SKILLS

Proven ability to interact on a positive note with people of different cultures and personality types. Multi-disciplinary team participation in the medical sector and business profession. Experience working with clients in healthcare settings, home settings, as well as within various types of business environment.

ORGANIZATIONAL SKILLS

Demonstrate time management in providing excellent care for multiple patients utilizing considerable nursing assessment and judgment while giving prescribed care. Extensive involvement in healthcare and the business industry collaborating with team players for positive outcome/productivity.

TEACHING

Experience in providing clients the necessary knowledge and information by utilizing varied and appropriate teaching methods to accommodate the different learning styles of the typical adult learner.

PROFESSIONAL EXPERIENCE

- Registered Nurse - **Medical Center, My Town,FL**
  March 2013 - present
  Health System, My Town, FL
  January 2008 – August 2012
  Health System, My Town, FL
  July 2006 – April 2008
- Home Health Aide- **Home Health, My Town, FL**
  February 2005 – July 2006
- PCA/Nursing Assoc-**Community Hospital, My Town, FL**
  July 2005 – June 2006
- Prod Coordinator/CSR-**Advertising, My Town, FL**
  November 2002 – January 2004
- Acct Executive/CSR-**Wherever, My Town, FL**
  February 2000 – March 2002

EDUCATION

My University - Anytown, FL

- Associate of Science in Nursing (highest honors)

Florida University- Anytown, FL

- B Sc in Graphic Arts Technology (summa cum laude)

My College - Anytown, FL

- Associate of Arts in Business Administration

REFERENCES

Available upon request

Whew, there is a lot of information in that resume example!

Although she did use the bold, underlined, and italicized techniques that I teach, the overall format is not ideal. There is too much wording, and not all of the margins are utilized to the fullest.

By simply changing the format, this resume can be made to look more streamlined and attention-grabbing.

Take a look at the "after" version, and keep in mind all that I changed for this example is the formatting. I intentionally only changed this one ingredient so you can realize how impactful one change in a single ingredient can be.

Below, you will notice how my changes to the formatting and layout makes the resume visually stand out in more appealing fashion.

Additionally, by fully utilizing the full right and left margins, using different font sizing, bold, underlined, and italicized fonts, the resume appropriately commands the attention of the reader.

Go ahead: take a peek and notice all of the strategic enhancements that have been made to the formatting and layout of this example.

OH MY GOODNESS
BS, RN

1234 NW Main Street, Anywhere, FL 33333

123.456.7890 OhMyGoodness@gmail.com

SUMMARY

Active Florida Registered Nurse licenses with over seven years experience working in the acute care setting, understanding the processes and workflow common in this environment; solid customer service background that includes excellent interpersonal skills and the ability to interact positively as part of a multi-disciplinary team. Possess strong critical thinking and decision-making abilities; highly analytical. Competent in managing multiple priorities and meeting deadlines. Excellent written and verbal communications skills. Experience working with various computer applications within the acute care setting, as well as the business sector. Comfortable working with the internet and technology. Looking for the opportunity to transition into Clinical Informatics.

QUALIFICATIONS

CUSTOMER SERVICE

Competent in communicating with internal and external customers, whether in person or by telephone to establish rapport, provide assistance, and recommend solutions. Accustomed to responding and resolving customer concerns, providing win-win resolutions in response to client inquiries. Responsible for company-client follow-up and liaison, which include timely reviews, proficient multi-tasking, and meeting tight deadlines.

INTERPERSONAL SKILLS

Proven ability to interact on a positive note with people of different cultures and personality types. Multidisciplinary team participation in the medical sector and business profession. Experience working with clients in healthcare settings and home settings, as well as within various types of business environments.

ORGANIZATIONAL SKILLS

Demonstrate time management in providing excellent care for multiple patients utilizing considerable nursing assessment and judgment while giving prescribed care. Extensive involvement in healthcare and the business industry, collaborating with team players for positive outcome/productivity.

TEACHING

Experience in providing clients the necessary knowledge and information by utilizing varied and appropriate teaching methods to accommodate the different learning styles of the typical adult learner.

PROFESSIONAL EXPERIENCE

Registered Nurse

Medical Center, My Town, FL 03/2013 – present

Health System, My Town, FL 01/2008 – 08/2012

Health System, My Town, FL 07/2006 – 04/2008

Home Health Aide

Home Health, My Town, FL 02/2005 – 07/2006

PCA/Nursing Associate

Community Hospital, My Town, FL 07/2005 – 06/2006

Prod Coordinator/CSR

Advertising, My Town, FL 11/2002 – 01/2004

Acct Executive/CSR

Wherever, My Town, FL 02/2000 – 03/2002

EDUCATION

My University - Anytown, FL

Associate of Science in Nursing (highest honors)

Florida University- Anytown, FL

B Sc in Graphic Arts Technology (summa cum laude)

My College - Anytown, FL

Associate of Arts in Business Administration

REFERENCES

Available upon request

Oh My Goodness, BS, RN

Did you notice how this version is visually more intriguing and commands the attention of the reader?

Just like the magazine cover, the "after" layout utilizes all of the margins: right, left, top, and bottom.

Right now, take the time to go to your resume and change the format. Step by step, ingredient by ingredient, you are making your resume a big bucks generator!

Remember, the first ingredient of a great resume is the format and layout.

Name and Initials

Reflect back to when you first learned how to cook and bake. It was very easy to misconstrue "tbsp" and "tsp," and yet the one extra letter made a big difference in the finished product: your outcome.

The initials are important on a resume too. By listing too many initials, or not enough of them, the outcome of your resume can be dramatically affected, just as it can be in cooking and baking.

What it comes down to is being specific about what initials do or don't make this kind of difference.

Not sure which is which?

Let's look at another example from a second nurse client of mine.

This time I am just going to focus in on the top portion of the resume, the name and initials.

WHY B. NORMAL

1234 Any Drive, My Town, AR
(123) 456-7890 ♦ Why2014@hotmail.com

Notice the format and layout. Remember, that is the first key ingredient.

Yes, the format and layout look amazing because of the right font, layout, and full use of margins. And yes, it commands that attention of the reader by making your eye read all of the information.

So what is the problem? Look again.

Reread it slowly.

Do you see the problem yet?

Don't feel bad if this problem is not jumping out at you. This common mistake is found all over the country in the resumes of both newly graduated and experienced RNs.

For the reader, the person who is looking for an RN, the name and appropriate initials are very important and need to be positioned immediately up front in the resume.

If the reader immediately sees that the person applying has the correct initials, and I do not mean middle name initials, then it drives them to read more of the resume.

Remember: we're talking "tbsp" versus "tsp." What is the difference? HUGE.

The same is true with the name and initials on a resume.

Look now.

WHY NORMAL, RN, BSN

1234 Any Drive, My Town, AR
(123) 456-7890 ♦ Why2014@hotmail.com

Do you notice the difference now?

Having not only "RN," but what type of RN (in this case BSN) right up front immediately affords the reader the insight that the person applying has what the reader is looking for in an applicant.

Additionally, enlarging the font size of the name makes it stand out more and again, fully commands the attention of the reader.

This is such a simple step, and yet it is so instrumental in having your resume get noticed.

If you doubt that something little like this makes a big difference, reflect back on the ramifications of not understanding the tiny difference of tbsp. and tsp. It truly changes the outcome.

Contact Info

Baking can be confusing. You first start with having to consistently note the difference between tbsp. and tsp. before you put the measured ingredients into the bowl.

Often, the directions are made easier when a recipe visually delineates tbsp. versus tsp. as "Tbs" versus "tsp." The capital 'T' really helps the person reading the recipe.

Guess what? The same is true with a resume.

If you visually change the size of the correct contact information on your resume, you make it far easier for the reader to get in touch with you.

SO HOPEFUL
123 Main Street, Anytown, CA 90210
Tel: (123) 456-7890
Email: sohopeful@unbc.ca

Look again at the above example. All of the contact information is in the same size font. Although this may seem trivial, it really is not.

Just as in baking, each ingredient, even if only a dash, pinch, or smidgen, makes a difference in the overall product.

Look at the smidgen that has been tweaked below.

Carmen Kosicek, RN, MSN

SO HOPEFUL
123 Main Street, Anytown, CA 90210
Tel: (123) 456-7890
Email: sohopeful@unbc.ca

Now do you see the difference?

The home address is not the important contact information nowadays, so make that font smaller. Seriously, no one will mail you a letter via snail mail anymore, nor show up at your house. These days, you will most likely receive an e-mail or a phone call from an interested potential employer.

With that being said, clearly the reader needs your telephone and email.

If you have a land line phone number and a cell phone number, use your cell phone number.

Why?

Do you really want anyone at your home answering a call from a potential employer to set up an interview other then you? Do you really want your home voice message to play for a potential employer?

More than likely, the answer to both of these questions is no. That is why you should list your cell phone number.

Additionally, be mindful of the outgoing voice message on your cell so that is friendly and appropriate for potential employers.

Now let's address your e-mail information.

If you are using a school e-mail address, change it immediately.

Why?

A school e-mail address showcases that you are a new grad and that may not work in your favor. I will go into this in further detail later when we examine a new grad resume in full.

Age discrimination happens based merely on resumes. Actually, there are multiple areas of insight on age discrimination so pay attention!

If you use an outdated e-mail address, such as one from AOL, you are showing your age. Heck, even MSN as an e-mail is considered older and begs an update.

Do you think I'm kidding?

Think about it.

My mother just turned seventy and she has an AOL email address. Honestly, I don't know of anyone in their fifties, forties, thirties, or twenties who still uses AOL. It feels like AOL e-mails came out back when dial-up internet was the norm!

A MSN e-mail is common for forty-year-olds and up.

No need to date yourself!

If you don't want to show your age and you have an outdated e-mail address, fix it!

If you are not sure what e-mail addresses are current, simply ask your twenty-year-old classmates, friends, your children, or your friends' children. They will be honest and they will know what is current.

See, it is all the little things that make a difference!

You may have noticed that other important ingredients were missing from the example above.

Did you catch this?

Correct. The initials!

So how would I recommend that you write your contact information? Take a look below.

SO HOPEFUL, RN, ADN

123 Main Street, Anytown, CA 90210

(123) 456-7890

sohopeful@gmail.com

As you can see, the name and appropriate initials are present, as well as set in a larger font size and bolded. The physical address is the smallest, because remember, no one is snail-mailing you information nor showing up at your door.

One phone number, preferably your cell, is listed along

with a current, updated e-mail address.

Skip your middle initial. If you have a hyphenated last name, only put the name that you most commonly go by. If that truly is the hyphenated name, then list it. Otherwise, simply list one last name.

As you're learning, attention to the details makes a huge difference. Look at it this way. In baking, you mainly use leveled, precisely measured ingredients. This step is yet another leveled, precisely strategic step in creating a big bucks resume.

Besides, using this technique makes the text clean and eye catching as well.

Summary

When you bake, the recipe normally tells you up front what the yield is for the final outcome. That way, you know if you will have enough of the final product for your needs. This step in the instructions is extremely helpful in that it allows you to know if your recipe should be doubled or tripled, or is fine as it is for the final amount you need to make and serve.

The same again is true for a big bucks resume.

Right up front, the reader needs to know in a strong statement why you are a good fit for the position. Finding someone who is a good fit is the final outcome they are looking to achieve.

Commonly, I see objective statements on healthcare resumes. This is an outdated mistake.

Clearly, everyone knows that your objective is to land the job that you are applying for, so skip that wasted step and replace it with a strong summary statement of your qualifications and skill set.

Let me be clear, I do not want you to list that you can start IVs, insert a foley, and pass meds. It is a given that any RN is competent in these entry-level skills.

Can you imagine if a bartender told you they mixed drinks, served up long necks, and even poured pop? You would already have in your mind that any bartender could do these things, because they are some of the most basic, entry-level skills that make up every bartender's job.

The same is true in a professional summary statement on a resume for a nurse.

There simply is no need to point out the obvious, showing that you are average, or suggesting that you only have the basic, entry-level skillset. And please, do not list in anyway that you are below average! I'm not kidding. I've actually seen that!

Instead, showcase your *above* average characteristics.

This is one of the most challenging aspects of a resume for most nurses. Why? Because relating the healthcare skillset to the business of healthcare has not usually been taught, and yet that is what is needed in today's healthcare landscape to secure the position you want.

Again, these are all real-life examples. I include them so that you can see what your competition (or in some cases, the lack of it) is like, and how to positively position yourself to win.

Here we go with a real "before" summary example:

PROFESSIONAL SUMMARY
Bilingual six year experienced Bachelorette prepared healthcare professional.

Other than learning that this applicant speaks another language, has nursing experience, and a bachelor's degree, nothing else stands out as to why this person should even be phoned for an interview.

Nothing showcases what type of worker this RN has been, let alone her past patient load and customer service outcomes.

Be aware that learning how to successfully write a big bucks resume takes time, work, and insight. Step by step, just as in baking, this is a process that can be learned, but it takes time.

After watching my free video series at http://carmenk.crystalcleardm.com/ , and reading about my take on making a resume stand out, this is what this same nurse came up with on her own.

PROFESSIONAL SUMMARY
Seeking a challenging position as a bilingual, experienced Registered Nurse within an organization searching for a diligent, responsible, and trustworthy professional that is willing to go the extra mile as a valued part of a collaborate effort in the positive growth of the company.

True, it is a bit stronger, but it still is not grabbing the reader and making them pick up the phone and schedule an interview.

Really look at the words and think of their impact, or lack of impact.

Wouldn't any organization want a responsible and trustworthy nurse? How about a nurse that would go the extra mile? You would expect the minimum requirement to be that the nurse collaborated in the effort of positive growth for the hospital, right?

See what I mean about not stating the obvious, or showcasing that you are average, or worse yet, below average?

With a summary statement like one in the example above, this resume will likely be tossed aside.

Think about this. If you were the recruiter, how would you position and explain a job-seeker who you thought was an especially strong candidate to the manager seeking to fill that job opening? Alternately, how would you as a recruiter describe a candidate who is only average?

These are the kinds of questions you need to ask yourself when you look at your own resume summary.

Try this on for speed:

PROFESSIONAL SUMMARY

Bilingual RN, BSN with six solid years of nursing insights and experiences at a nationally recognized Level 1 trauma center on a fast paced, cardiac step-down unit, rich with experiences blended in healthcare, business, marketing and management, presently seeking an innovative and progressive position which will afford opportunities to enhance medically infused technologically insights to further decrease healthcare spending while continuing to meet or exceed state and federal guidelines and drive key providers the ability to enhance healthcare standards within the local community.

BAM!

Yes, the phone will likely be picked up with this summary statement and the applicant phoned for an interview.

Why?

Right away, the reader knows that this is a RN, BSN who is bilingual. Additionally, the reader recognizes what type of facility the RN has gleaned insights from—a nationally recognized Level 1 trauma center.

This alone paints quite the positive picture for the recruiter.

Wouldn't you agree?

Don't worry if you don't speak multiple languages, or if you have not worked at a Level 1 trauma center. Your insights from long-term care, home health, occupational health, and more are reasons to proudly wave your own flag.

Painting the picture appropriately is the key. Really describe the working environment, conditions, your impact, and most importantly, the outcomes from your impact. This is the way to blend the business of healthcare for today's times.

Stop and reread that last paragraph.

Why? So many times I see nurses who do not realize that what they are doing at their jobs, their everyday routine, is actually a big deal.

I'm not talking only about actual job performance. Rather, I'm suggesting that what is needed is for you to fully describe, in depth, exactly what a nurse like you does on the front lines of the job.

Let me make this really clear.

Part of what you do is cost containment.

Although this sounds like a fancy business term, it is actually a real-life example that nurses, no matter what facet of nursing they work within, are doing every day.

You may be puzzled when first presented with this idea, trying to picture cost containment within the context of nursing. Here is just one example. I'll bet you're used to having to run to the Pixis for any and all supplies, while being cognizant of how many supplies you pull as you strive to use the least amount of only what is truly required for a particular task or procedure.

Sounds familiar, right? Doing more with less.

This is one example of cost containment in nursing.

Here's another example. The charge nurse looks at the clock, guesstimating if the current nursing staff is able to take on the increasing patient load, along with the higher census at present, and if the current nursing staff is able to carry the acuity load demands of the patients.

The charge nurse calculates whether the patient load can continue to be carried by the current staff until the upcoming change of shift nurses come in, because the alternative option would be to call in the on-call nurse, and that would negatively add to the overall staffing budget.

Again, it's a case of doing more and more with less and less to contain costs.

Even experiences that are not in healthcare count if highlighted in such a positive manner.

Think about it.

If you have worked at McDonald's, that is something to brag about!

Why?

Well, to start with, McDonald's is a Fortune 500 company and is even recognized internationally. Compare that to your local hospital. Even if it is a biggie, it is not a Fortune 500 company, and more than likely it is not internationally recognized.

McDonald's has fabulous customer service and, clearly, all of their employees have strategic training in this arena.

If you don't already know, hospitals are moving more and more towards higher levels of customer service in addition to their healthcare insights and outcomes.

So again, the key is to learn how to word your experiences so that they will capture the skillset you have gleaned from past positions and translate these to the current position you are seeking.

This is where resume insights are required above and beyond simple cookie-cutter formulas.

Everyone comes with a different set of experiences and seeking unique positions as a nurse. Therefore, a nursing resume is simply not something that works as a one-size-fits-all.

The blend of business with healthcare is what is needed in nursing today for nurses to have the numerous doors of opportunities open to them.

To be clear, the doors of opportunity are already flying open for nurses who present themselves with the right blend of healthcare and business. If this was not true, the standard healthcare resume that you were taught in school would be working, and you would be landing positions inside and outside of traditional nursing. But that is not happening.

Again, traditional nursing resumes, the kind that the colleges continue to incorrectly promote as best practice, are not leading to opportunities that result in nursing employment. Those outdated resumes are not helping nurses in 2014 and beyond. Nurses, from the newly graduated to the experienced, are not hearing their phones ring with interview offers when using these antiquated nursing resumes.

Instead, nurses often state that they are stuck in their career path and falsely believe they need to add on more and more pieces of paper in order to move up in their nursing careers.

Based on my work with the thousands of nurses I've helped nationally with their resumes, interviewing techniques, salary negotiations, and more, this is not what I've experienced.

The nurses I've helped have learned that their experiences truly are a blend of business and healthcare. Once they learn how to showcase themselves appropriately within the business of healthcare, only then do they realize the many doors of opportunities there for them.

As I've mentioned, it takes a lot of time to put together a big bucks resume. Reflect back as to how long it took you to become a nurse. You did not simply read a book and suddenly you were functioning as a nurse.

Nor did you simply go to the simulation lab after watching the videos, practicing on the manikin, and then become an expert at foley catheter insertion on your first solo try. It helped if you had guidance from someone who had experience, and even then, it took practice on your part. Big bucks resume writing is no different.

Experience

When you bake, the directions are detailed even down to the baking temperature variations for different altitudes.

Again, the same is true for the makings of a big bucks resume for nurses.

All of the important details need to be present on your resume to showcase how you, the candidate, are not only a perfect match, but how you are the perfect candidate who has proven experience, in any field, to make a positive impact.

You need to be detailed in your approach and cover the different variations of skillset transfer that an employer will be looking for. This will aid in the effectiveness a candidate is seen to likely bring for a particular position.

Additionally, you need to make sure that your resume covers any relevant search engine optimization keywords simply to make it past the computer scanner. Highlight your outcomes and results, and have your resume get passed on to an actual human!

Just as with the experience summary, this is neither the time nor place to showcase your skills. Rather, this is the time and place to showcase your skillset and the impact you have made.

Remember, you don't need to list that you can start IVs, as that is simply a skill. Rather, you need to showcase your skillset—meaning how your impact of starting IVs leads to decreased prep time in the pre-surgical area, etc.

Why do you need to do this?

Describing your impact is crucial, because the healthcare environment is now the business of healthcare. And in business, it is about what you have done, how well you have done it, and the impact your results have made for the company.

Describing your impact will allow a new potential employer to see the positive impact you will potentially have in their company.

Although the business of healthcare is the focus, the vast majority of healthcare resumes are not up to par. Sadly, there are numerous companies literally waiting for a candidate who understands the business of healthcare to apply, and nursing knowledge is utilized across an array of fields.

Are you not doing this? No wonder your phone is not ringing with opportunities!

Here is a look at another one of the resumes floating around in the current marketplace. Although a college may have told this nurse her resume is good, I disagree. Then again, I am shooting for a big bucks resume.

Here's a quick revisit to our big bucks resume ingredient list:

- Format and layout
- Name and initials
- Contact info

- Summary
- Experience
- Education

The experience ingredient is your main core. There are a lot of areas that you will need to go over with a fine-tooth comb, so I will address them one by one after you review the real-life resume example below.

<u>**PROFESSIONAL EXPERIENCE**</u>
Health Care Center – My Town, CA
03/2009 – PRESENT
Nurse Supervisor/ADON

- ***Responsible*** for the overall direction, management and evaluation of nursing care to all residents.
- ***Perform*** registered nurse duties as a Nurse Supervisor, which included primary planning, organizing, and evaluating care for residents requiring complex medical attention.
- ***Consult*** with physicians and other various healthcare clinicians as the Coordinator of care.
- ***Manage*** the deliverance of IV infusion therapy, analyze lab results, and administer medication.
- ***Worked*** as treatment nurse, a position requiring side-by-side collaboration with wound specialist.

Another Care Center – My Town, CA
February, 2003 – Oct, 2008
Registered Nurse/License Practical Nurse/Certified Nurse Assistant

- ***Provided*** healthcare services to patients with chronic physical or mental disorders as Nurse Supervisor.
- ***Facilitated*** routine blood draws, analyzed lab results, and administration of medication as primary Care Manager.
- ***Documented*** all necessary elements of the nursing assessment treatments, medications, discharge instructions, and follow up care.

So many areas to fix!

Okay. To begin, let's look first at the easiest fix: the dates. Think back to our discussion of format and layout.

Nurses need to pay attention to detail at work, and therefore, a nurse should pay attention to detail on his or her resume as well.

In the example above, look at the inconsistencies in the way the date is formatted alone. Being consistent is a must! Additionally, using the XX/XXXX format is recommended instead of spelling out the date.

Why?

This is easier on the eye, visually more congruent, and most importantly, the computer scanner, who will view your resume first, prefers dates in the numerical format.

It is best to stick with two to four bullet points for each job. Remember, the goal of the resume is to make your phone ring, not to tell the reader everything. Your goal is to intrigue the reader so that he or she wants to call you for an interview and learn more.

When you limit yourself to between two to four bullet points, you must make each point strong, showcasing what you have done and how well you have done it and what your impact was to the company.

If you point out the obvious or showcase that you are average, you have wasted space on your resume and your phone will likely not ring.

Look at the example above again. Everything listed there is really showcasing that this nurse has met the average need of the position.

I do not see how this person has demonstrated their effectiveness in their position, let alone anything about their positive impact on the job for the company.

Instead, every bullet point listed is something obvious. So you don't have to keep flipping back, here again are the first two bullet points:

- ***Responsible*** for the overall direction, management and evaluation of nursing care to all residents.
- ***Perform*** registered nurse duties as a Nurse Supervisor, which included primary planning, organizing, and evaluating care for residents requiring complex medical attention.

Again, isn't every nurse responsible for the direction and evaluation of nursing care to residents? Really! There is nothing in this bullet-pointed list about how many residents or anything else specific. It really is so loosely and generally written that it could be about anyone performing this job role.

Again, if you were the nursing recruiter, how would you explain this candidate to the hiring manager in two minutes as someone being above and beyond, someone who stands out and is worthy of an interview?

You can't. Because you haven't been given the kind of information that shows this.

If I was the recruiter trying to sell this potential candidate to the manager, I would be hard-pressed to do so.

So how would I recommend making this section of your resume different, to make it stand out and to increase the chances of having your phone ring?

By blending healthcare with business, because again, nowadays, nursing is the business of healthcare.

Here is an example of how to improve on the last sample resume.

PROFESSIONAL EXPERIENCE

Health Care Center – My Town, CA 03/2009 – PRESENT

Assistant Director of Nursing

- ***Responsible*** for the direction, management and evaluation of nursing care to 120 orthopedic residents, implementing innovative hiring, training and retention methods of healthcare staffing, resulting in decreased turnover rates by 35% in the first 12 months, far surpassing exceeding corporate expectations.
- ***Perform*** supervisory duties with attention to cultural differences across an array of ethnicities from clients to staff, leading to an enhanced respect for differences and similarities of cultures, thereby forming stronger working relationships amongst staff leading to increased staff retention of 25%, and increased referrals from satisfied clients by 15% annually.
- ***Consult*** across a mixed healthcare team, focusing on transparent communication, thereby streamlining plan of care meeting and exceeding healthcare performance outcome goals by 10% within the first six months of implementation along with decreased readmission rates by 5%.

These bullets are stronger because they vividly describe a more focused picture of what the candidate achieved in his or her current position.

The potential new employer can now clearly see the candidate's capabilities and how he or she can make a difference in the position they are applying for within the new organization.

And what is the outcome of this change? You guessed it. A resume showcasing results leads to interviews.

Appropriately highlighting the experience section of a resume is not something that works with cookie-cutter format. Rather, the experience and summary areas of a well-appointed resume must be focused on showcasing what you have done and the impactful results you had while doing it.

These two areas, experience and summary, will be unique to each individual, and rightfully so. This is precisely why I will not show example after example of "after" resumes. I've found that when multiple examples are given, many people will simply copy them, and then expect the stellar results that I speak of.

If you want these kinds of results, you first have to do the work.

But how do you best do that?

Before you attempt to express the intricate details of your experience, first visualize the bigger picture. Work backwards, finding the words to capture that bigger picture and then work on best showcasing how you arrived at the ultimate outcome.

Just as when you're baking, you first look at the bigger picture: the outcome or final product. Seriously, think about how often you admire a picture of the final product and then determine, based on how good it looks, that you want to make and enjoy it yourself.

From there, most people will briefly read the ingredients list, but they hone in on the intricate details of the process needed to make the final product.

To create a big bucks resume, replicate this process when writing about your experience.

Education

The last ingredient for a big bucks resume is appropriately showcasing your education.

Listing your education is the icing on the cake. Clearly, you have the required education for the position you have applied for. What you need to do is to frame this information appropriately on your resume.

Do be cognizant of the fact that there is a difference between required and preferred educational requirements.

Required means that it is a must-have. Preferred means that you do not have to have the degree or experience stated, but they would like or prefer for you to have it.

Here is and example of how *not* to showcase your education:

EDUCATION
2012 Bachelor of Science Degree RN-BSN
Chamberlain College of Nursing, Naperville, IL
June 2012 **GPA 3.919**

2008 Associate of Arts' Degree in Nursing
Seward County Community College, Liberal, KS
GPA 3.7
Magna Cum Laude

So why is this not a good way to do this?

Remember, the number one ingredient: format and layout. First off, the educational information listed above is visually challenging for the reader.

Look at it.

You really have to read every line to decipher necessary information.

Another problematic area is the year. It is not important *when* you graduated from college, but rather *that* you graduated from college. By putting the year on there, you are opening yourself up to age discriminatory practices.

How?

Think about it. If you saw that the person's education was an associate's degree in 2008, you would assume, more than likely, that the person graduated from high school in 2006, because getting an associate's degree is typically a two-year process.

The problem here is that perhaps this person was thirty-two or fifty-two when they went to junior college, and now the reader assumes that the applicant is in their early twenties. Perhaps the employer wants someone older for the job.

So what happens next?

You guessed it. The resume would get tossed.

Again, there is no need to give out information that is not needed.

To test this theory, think about your healthcare provider, nurse practitioner, or physician. Do you know *when* he or she graduated or do you know *that* he or she graduated? See what I mean?

Okay, here is a good attempt at how to showcase your education with a much better format and layout:

EDUCATION
Chamberlain College of Nursing, Naperville, IL
Bachelor of Science in Nursing
GPA 3.919, Presidential Honor Graduate

Seward County Community College, Liberal, KS
Associate of Science in Nursing
GPA 3.72, Magna Cum Laude

This is still not as spot on as it could be. Below is how I would recommend that you highlight your education on a resume:

EDUCATION
Chamberlain College of Nursing, Naperville, IL
Bachelor of Science in Nursing
GPA 3.92

Seward County Community College, Liberal, KS
Associate of Science in Nursing
GPA 3.72

What is the difference, and why do I recommend these slight but impactful differences?

The format and layout have been tweaked here even more by making the font size strategically smaller and larger so that, visually, the most important information commands the attention of the reader.

Look at it again.

BEFORE:

EDUCATION
Chamberlain College of Nursing, Naperville, IL
Bachelor of Science in Nursing
GPA 3.919, Presidential Honor Graduate

Seward County Community College, Liberal, KS
Associate of Science in Nursing
GPA 3.72, Magna Cum Laude

AFTER:

EDUCATION
Chamberlain College of Nursing, Naperville, IL
Bachelor of Science in Nursing
GPA 3.92

Seward County Community College, Liberal, KS
Associate of Science in Nursing
GPA 3.72

On the "after" version above, it's easier to notice the degrees that the candidate has earned first, and then the school. But you don't waste time focusing on where the college was located, as that portion is immaterial.

Why did I take off the original information listed after the GPA?

With GPAs of 3.70 or higher, it is assumed that honors status has been achieved. Thus, removing the name of the award will allow more attention to be focused on the GPA itself.

Again, think about your provider. A provider will say where he or she went to college and what his or her degree is in, but he or she does not typically go on to state their collegiate educational awards.

Yes, you worked hard for a solid and strong GPA, and yes, you should be proud of it. Stating the strong GPA of 3.70 or higher will showcase a historical track record of education excellence and historical learning pattern, and yes, it is a great idea to have this on a resume.

However, if your GPA is not 3.70 or higher, it is not recommended to include it on your resume. Remember, you do not want to appear average or close to average; you want to be desirable by looking above average.

If you are new in your career, the educational section should be towards the top of your resume, after your summary statement.

However, if you are experienced in your career, the educational section should be at the end of your resume, after the professional experience section.

Why?

If you are experienced, a potential new employer realizes that you have the required degrees and is more interested in what you have done with your degree than the fact that you have it.

They're looking to understand the experiences you have had, how you have made a positive impact for the companies that you have worked for, and how you can potentially help their company.

Let's go back to our baking metaphor. When you are baking, your final product may not look exactly like the image of the product you wanted to bake. This is because your final product is unique to the temperature of your oven, your elevation, and other specific factors.

Likewise, your resume may not look exactly like these examples here, but overall, it should be similar. Your resume will be unique to you and your experiences, just as your baked goods will take shape relative the picture in the cookbook, by way of your oven temperature and elevation.

Overall though, when you implement these techniques, the outcome should be a big bucks resume!

Attention grabbing—that is the key! Next, we will address how to make sure your big bucks resume commands the attention of everyone who reads it.

CHAPTER 4: How to Write an Attention-Grabbing Big Bucks Resume

Movie trailers. They grab your attention, showcase just the right amount of details from key scenes, and leave you wanting to see the whole film. Or at least, that's what a good movie trailer does.

On the other hand, there are also movie trailers that showcase every best moment of the entire movie. Those drive me insane!

Movie trailers that grab my attention and drive me to want to see the rest of the story have a tendency to steer me towards movies I enjoy—the kind that make you feel like you've spent your time and money well.

That all starts with a well put together trailer that grabs my attention and draws my interest.

Is your resume a good trailer for a great movie? It should be. Even if you are a new grad, you can make your resume great.

Is it great, though? Is it eye-catching?

Will this resume grab a reader's attention and drive him or her to view the resume in its entirety?

Will the reader feel that this resume was worth reading,

worth his or her time, and make him or her want to learn more about you?

Will the reader talk about how great this resume is after he or she has read it?

Keep reading, use the techniques I'm teaching you, and you bet they will!

In this chapter, we'll look at some of the big bucks techniques you can use to land your resume at the top of the stack, get the interview, and land the job!

New Grad RN Resumes

Lopa, a new grad in the Northeast, reached out to me after repeatedly applying for jobs soon after attaining her BSN. Yes, she had done the "spray and pray" method, and in doing so, had inadvertently tainted her own marketplace.

Although Lopa had passed her NCLEX, she could not break through the barrier of "New grads need not apply" or "No experience? No need to apply."

But everyone needs to gain experience somehow.

After taking less than one minute to review her resume, I could easily see why she was not making it past the online application, where the computer scanners were deciding whether her resume was worthy enough to be read by a real person.

Getting past the online job application system is a crucial first step that Lopa wasn't successfully reaching.
Like so many nurses, Lopa was playing a game without understanding its rules—the online application game.

However, that was only the start of Lopa's resume problems.

Why?

Well heck, even if a human had read it, there was no way she would be interviewed!

Take a look and see if you are now able to decipher what key ingredients are either in or are missing from Lopa's "before" resume.

As a reminder, here are the ingredients required for a successful big bucks resume:

- Format and layout
- Name and initials
- Contact info
- Summary
- Experience
- Education

L O P A   K A N D Y
BSN, RN
123 Main Street, Your Town, PA 90210
C: (123)-456-7890 (E): lkandy@students.jjc.edu

OBJECTIVE: To obtain a clinical nurse II position at Pennsylvania Hospital

LICENSURE/CERTIFICATION

Pennsylvania State Registered Nurse License: Active
AHA Basic Cardiac Life Support

EDUCATION

Your State University - Your Town, PA, 2009-2013

Bachelor of Science in Nursing – GPA 3.82
Summa Cum Laude

CLINICAL EXPERIENCE

Nursing Foundations- Long-Term Care, Capitol Healthcare Services (65 hours), Your Town, PA
Mental Health Nursing- Long-Term facility, So & So Psychiatric Center (70hours), Your Town, PA
NUR I - Med-Surge Unit-3 West, ABC Hospital (84 hours), Your Town, PA
NUR II- Med-Surge Unit-3 East, ABC Hospital (75 hours), Your Town, PA
NUR III- Intermediate Care Unit- ABC Hospital (100 hours), Your Town, PA
Community Health Nursing- Home Health Care, ABC Hospice (70 hours), Your Town, PA
Maternal/Newborn Health- Maternity/Labor &Delivery, Community Care (70 hours), Your Town, PA
Pediatric PACU/NICU, ABC Hospital (12 hours), Your Town, PA

WORK EXPERIENCE

Registered Nurse, Adult Day Center, Your Town, PA. Conduct health assessments, implement care plans, document patient care, and revise care plan as necessary (11/2013-present).

Peer Tutor, Your State University Academic Enrichment Center, Your Town, PA. Teaching level 2 and 3 nursing and support courses (03/2012-04/2012)

Student Worker, Research Program, Your Town, PA. Assisted in maintaining documents and records and creating new data file with a high level of efficiency and accuracy (06/2011-08/2011)

Student Researcher, Summer Research Internships, Your Town, PA.
Experienced to conduct a genomic study in model organism, *C. elegans* (06/2010-07/2010)

COMMUNITY INVOLVEMENT
Southern Go Red for Women – Health screening- Your Town, PA - 2013
Community Health Fair- Poster Presentation- Your Town, PA- 2012
Annual Culture Day- Cultural Liaison – Your Town, PA- Spring 2012 & 2013
38th Anniversary of Honor's Day- Scientific Research Presentation- Your Town, PA- 2011

AWARDS / HONORS

Academic Excellence Award	2010 - 2011, 2011 - 2012
Certificate of Professional Development	2013
Nursing Honors Society, Inductee	2013
State Nursing Scholarship recipient	2011 - 2012
President's list	2009 - 2011, Spring 2012 & 2013
Dean's List	Fall 2011, Fall 2012
Student Nurses Association, Member	2011 - Present

Changes

So what did you see in Lopa's resume that you now know to change?

A lot! Right?

Look again at the "before" resume this time as if you were a potential employer.

Go through the ingredient list and make notes of your insights about how each one is either working or not working in this resume.

- Format and layout
- Name and initials
- Contact info
- Summary

- Experience
- Education

Really think about what you have learned thus far. What could be enhanced, added, or removed?

Now that we've discussed each ingredient of a big bucks resume, along with the rationale for each one, I want to challenge you to enhance your learning. You can do this by going back over each ingredient in depth.

This will solidify what you have learned so far and tap not just into the different learning styles, but into the different memory recall sections in your brain to drive your learning.

Remember, it takes time to learn a new way of doing anything.

In nursing school, you did not learn a new-to-you clinical skill by simply reading the book or watching a video. You first had to learn the skill from reading, then watching a video perhaps and later by practicing the skill in the simulation or skill lab. You then gradually gained confidence as you integrated new-to-you concepts when treating your first patients as a student nurse and later as a nurse. The learning process takes time.

Writing a big bucks resume is no different.

To highlight this further, I want you to see what happened next in Lopa's story.

After Lopa watched my free video series at

http://carmenk.crystalcleardm.com/, she reached out to me and we spoke about my recommendations for what she should do differently on her resume.

Remember, learning takes time. And writing a big bucks resume is a learning process.

Here is Lopa's attempt at a big bucks resume. Again, here she is in the learning process, so you will note that many of the ingredients are still not spot on or even present at all.

LOPA KANDY, RN, BSN
123 Main Street
(C): 123-456-7890
Your Town, PA 19803
(E): lkandy@students.jjc.edu

OBJECTIVE: Quadrilingual, Bachelor's-prepared RN looking for a full-time staff nurse position in acute-care settings

EDUCATION & CREDENTIALS:

Bachelor of Science in Nursing, May 2013 GPA 3.82
Your University - Your Town, PA
Summa Cum Laude

Your State Registered Nurse License, *Active*
American Heart Association BCLS certified, *Expires 08/2015*

WORK EXPERIENCES:

Registered Nurse, Adult Day Center, Your Town, PA 11/2013- Present

- Conducted initial health assessments of participants to evaluate patient's needs, developed care plans, implement participant care plans and record progress, ensure safe medication administration, and revise care plan as necessary.
- Collaborated with multidisciplinary team regarding the provision of the participant's healthcare

Supplemental Instruction Leaders, Your State University, Your Town, PA Spring 2012

- Taught level 2 and 3 nursing courses to students enrolled in Academic Support Center
- Assisted students in developing study strategies and critical thinking skills
- Demonstrated for excellence in teaching and coaching abilities

Student Worker, MBRS- RISE Research Scholars Program, Your Town, PA Summer 2011

- Responsible for lab supplies inventory, operating office

equipment and documenting data collection into database programs, organizing lab meeting, providing customer service

- Organized lab equipments and chemical kits to ensure proper storage and care
- Cited for excellence in interpersonal communications, teamwork, flexibility and reliability

Research Intern, NIH-RISE Summer Research Internship, Your Town, PA Summer 2010

- Conducted independent genomic research on model organism, *C.elegans* to study the role of genes in different stages of cell cycle
- Demonstrated talent for identifying key issues in research topics and analyzing collected data to further solve the problems.

COMMUNITY INVOLVEMENT & ACTIVITIES:

LOPA KANDY, RN, BSN

Southern Go Red for Women–Blood pressure and stroke evaluation- Your Town, PA-2013
Community Health Fair- Health teaching on obesity and nutrition- Your Town, PA- 2012
Annual Culture Day- Cultural Liaison of DSU- Your Town, PA- 2012 and 2013
Town Pointe Elementary school-Health screening and teaching-Your Town, PA-2012
38th Anniversary of Honors Day- Scientific Research Oral Presentation- Your Town, PA-2011

SKILLS:

- MS Word, MS Excel, MS PowerPoint, Adobe Acrobat, HTML, Windows 8, Windows 7, XP
- EHR software: McKesson and Millennium Pharmacy systems
- Languages – English, Hindi, Gujarati, Urdu

AWARDS & HONORS:

Academic Excellence Award	2010-2011 and 2011–2012
Nursing Honors Society, Inductee	2013

President's list	2009 – 2011, Spring 2012 & 2013
Dean's List	Fall 2011 & Fall 2012
Student Nurses Association, Member	2011-present
State Nursing Scholarship, recipient	2011-2012

Clearly, Lopa is on a learning curve and headed in the right direction. After learning from the insights highlighted in this book, you too will be on the learning curve headed in the right direction for your own big bucks resume.

In reviewing this newer version of her resume, you most likely noticed that Lopa made a lot of positive progress such as changing the font size, implementing bold, underlined, and italic techniques, and even maximizing the margins. This is all well done, and really adds to the resume's visual appeal.

However, in my opinion, Lopa's revamped resume will not get her noticed.

Why is this?

Did you notice any key ingredients missing? And similarly, did you see any of the unnecessary ingredients we talked about earlier that can lend themselves to discriminatory hiring practices?

If you did, great job! If not, try going back through both the revamped resume and your checklist again. Make notes on what you find to further enhance your learning.

We'll discuss Lopa's resume further a little deeper into this chapter, but first let's revisit some of what we have already learned about the importance of using a big bucks resume when applying for nursing positions.

Why is there such a push to nail this big bucks resume?

As we discussed in an earlier chapter, applying with an ineffective resume will not make your phone ring with opportunities. And for every month that passes without landing the job you're seeking, that is costing you more than $4,300 a month!

Did you forget how that amount was calculated?

The national average pay for a new grad RN is $25 per hour. With fifty-two weeks in a year, working forty hours a week equates to 2080 total working hours in a year. Two weeks of vacation is standard but that is paid vacation, so it will not alter the calculations. Based on this, with full-time hours of 2080 x $25 per hour, that equates to $52,000 a year or $4,333.33 a month.

Lastly, every semester and every quarter, nursing schools are cranking out more and more new RN grads. This flood of new grads is deadly to anyone who has not yet secured gainful employment, as employers will negatively view as undesirable those who graduated before the next, new class, and have yet to secure a position.

Rather than hiring whoever is left in the existing market, these employers often choose to wait for the cream of the crop from the next group of RN grads that comes every year like clockwork.

Don't forget, applying with an ineffective resume, in

addition to not getting you noticed, also negatively taints the market you are desperately seeking to land a position within. Your data is captured and the computer will recall that you were not the best candidate in the past, for whatever reason.

What would magically change in a year from now?

Not much.

Thus, it is imperative to apply with a big bucks resume to shift the odds in your favor for the best opportunities available.

There is a lot on the line here, and time is of the essence.

How You Learned in School

Think about it. You did not learn how to catheterize someone simply by watching the video.

Instead, you watched the video that was thirty minutes or more in length, and then you practiced in the simulation or skills lab with an instructor.

You went on to practice this new technique with a group of colleagues until you felt confident enough to be checked off in the simulation or skills lab by the instructor. And yet with all that practice, when it was time to catheterize a real person, you still had your instructor help you.

Why would a resume be any different?

Why would you try it on your own when there is so much at stake?

True, you may take an online seminar like Lopa did before she reached out to me, or you may have looked at examples of other resumes that you found online or through your school. But you were not getting the results you wanted from someone who helps others, wouldn't you reach out for help from a new source?

Wouldn't you go to someone who has a track record of success by doing different things in nursing?

I know I would.

Online Application

The online application has changed the landscape of applying for nursing positions, or any position really—especially in a flooded market where volumes of people are vying for the same job opportunity.

Heed my warning, however: do not taint your market with the spray and pray method of putting your resume all over the place. Instead, be strategic in your approach with the guidance of someone who knows what they are doing.

Now, back to Lopa's resume. In order for her to truly be noticed in the competitive new grad job market in her area, Lopa's resume should reflect the business of healthcare.

This is what I did with Lopa's resume.

LOPA KANDY

RN, BSN

YOUR TOWN, PA 90210
PHONE 123-456-7890 • E-MAIL
CHANGE@GMAIL.COM

SUMMARY

Quadralingual BNS-RN. Responsible, compassionate, and dedicated healthcare professional with a strong background of customer service, critical thinking skills and pharmaceutical sales experience seeking enhanced career opportunities.

EDUCATION AND LICENSURE

Your State University – Your Town, PA
Bachelor of Science in Nursing
Summa Cum Laude

Licensure – **Registered Nurse, Compact State Multi License**

EXPERIENCE

Adult Day Center – Your Town, PA **11/2013 - Present**

Registered Nurse

- Successful utilization of critical thinking skills in organizing and prioritizing the care of patients, including dementia patients.
- Daily collaboration with multidisciplinary team regarding the provisions of the participants' healthcare, resulting in decreased spending of healthcare dollars per patient with outcomes far surpassing corporate expectations.

Biotech Company – PA **01/2014 – Present**

Clinical Sales Nurse Educator

- Charged with educational launch of a pharmacogenetic cutting edge technology, educating a various mix of physician practices from primary care to specialty MDs in Pain, Urology, Cardiac, OB, and beyond.
- Independent self-starter resulting in territory sales exceeding quota by 17% in the first six months.

CERTIFICATIONS, SKILLS, AND MEMBERSHIPS

- **American Heart Association Healthcare Provider CPR – BLS**
- **RN Compact State Multi-License**

NURSING INFORMATICS

- **McKesson**
- **Millennium Pharmacy Systems**

LANGUAGES

- **Hindi**
- **Urdu**
- **Gujarati**
- **English**

Compare

There are clearly numerous changes that I made. Go back and compare this version of Lopa's resume to the last one, line by line. Don't miss anything.

Reeking of New Grad

I do not want Lopa's resume, nor any new grad's resume, to reek of "new grad," so I took out the vast majority of school references, including the school-related e-mail address.

Do you want to hear something crazy?

Lopa's collegiate instructor specifically told her that the school e-mail looked more professional. Am I kidding? Nope, I cannot make this stuff up.

This is yet another example of how outdated the advice is from many nurses and, sadly, also many nursing instructors and even the career counselors in most colleges.

Now, I would actually agree with this advice if Lopa's e-mail was something like "partyanimal@gmail.com" or "momof3@gmail.com" and it was horrifically hard to get a new email address, but this was not the case in either regard.

A school e-mail looks professional if you are the instructor, but it reeks of "new grad" if you are not.

Times have changed. And that means it's time to get real! When it clearly doesn't work, why would you continue to listen to this outdated way of doing things?

Remove Clinicals

New grads across the country are being told to include their clinical rotations on their resume. I firmly believe this is a bad idea.

Why?

In each state, the Board of Nursing (BON) approves schools, colleges, and universities to run nursing programs. So each state's BON is the governing body of every nursing program in that entire state, setting the requirements for how many hours a nursing student must have in any particular clinical setting.

What this means for you is that if you are a new grad and you simply list your clinical experience, you're making yourself look exactly the same as every other nursing grad in your state. The only difference between the experience listed on your resume and everyone else's would be the location where you completed those hours.

Be mindful that the location is not always something to brag about.

Pecking Order

When it comes to the need to gain experience, it's important to look at your situation realistically. For instance, let's say you are in the Chicago area market and you did your rotations at one of the huge tertiary care hospitals there, like Northwestern, Rush, or Loyola. All of these hospitals have medical residents. And those residents are the first in the pecking order to get to do procedures—not the nursing students.

We're just keeping it real here. It's important to be aware of this.

There is a pecking order in life, and in the healthcare

world, doctors are at the top. This means they get first crack at the hands-on experience when the choice is between giving a procedure to a student doctor versus a student nurse. Heck, this is the case even if this scenario plays out between a student doctor versus an experienced nurse!

How does being aware of this help you?

Think about what happens if you have your nursing clinical rotations at a huge tertiary care hospital and then turn around and apply at a suburban hospital. Should you really list your clinical experience from the big, downtown hospitals? The suburban hospital will say that you *saw* a lot, but did not get to actually *do* a lot—because everyone knows that the medical residents get first dibs in the pecking order.

You see, the suburban hospital more than likely does not have medical residents. What's more, the suburban hospital employees understand how the pecking order works, and who gets the real experience.

For this reason, the suburban hospital is likely to turn their nose up at your application, because they need an RN who can function without an MD around.

Now let's think of this in reverse. If you did your clinical rotations in a suburban hospital setting and you are trying to land a job in the big, downtown hospitals, what they will notice is that you got your initial experience at one of the places where the "train wreck" cases from those outlying areas are regularly sent from to their huge tertiary downtown hospitals for specialized care.

This is true. Suburban hospitals do ship their challenging patients to the big tertiary care centers.

You see what I mean about the drawbacks of listing this kind of experience on your resume? No matter what way you list it, listing your nursing school clinical experiences is no longer advantageous to a new grad for the reasons I've discussed here. Perhaps it was different back in the day, but that is no longer the case in 2014 and beyond.

If a new grad implements this outdated resume technique, it simply waves the red flag even more that the fact that the RN is new to begin with. That can come back to haunt him or her.

The last thing you want is the person looking at your resume to assume that, based on a cursory glance at the information you have provided, you haven't learned enough. Whatever way you shake it, listing your clinical experience on your resume lends itself to this unfortunate outcome.

Stop giving recruiters and hiring managers reasons to not choose you.

Stop sending up the red flags on your resume that fly high and scream to the reader you are new, new, new.

Instead, highlight how much experience you do have in any role and frame it using the verbiage of the business of healthcare.

Results

So now that we've taken Lopa's resume through multiple steps of improvement, I bet what you're wondering is did the new, big bucks version work?

Well, yes. It did work!

Sure enough, once she began circulating the improved, big bucks version of her resume that I helped her with, Lopa—a new grad RN—did land a position as a Clinical Sales Nurse Educator at a Biotech company.

Although I firmly believe that any new grad needs a good two or more years of clinical nursing, I also believe that landing *any* position in nursing is by far better than landing a position outside of the field of nursing. Working in nursing, you get to start paying off student loan debt and increase your base of experience as a nurse.

Additionally, by building her base of experience in different facets of nursing, this technique will help Lopa to land a clinical nursing job without looking as if she has zero experience in nursing—and that is exactly what Lopa went on to do six months later.

The Bubble

The sad truth is that nursing exists in a bubble. Our profession is overwhelmingly antiquated in its tactics around how jobs are defined and worked.

Again, I am not against traditional nursing employment

venues—I am just showing you what really is going on outside of traditional nursing employment venues, and all the amazing opportunities that are out there and available to you if you're willing to look outside the bubble.

Think about this fact, big businesses are often financially incentivized by the federal government to hire a diverse workforce. A diverse workforce that incorporates more minorities.

At many of these companies, women fall into the minority category. Think about this. Women continue to dominate the nursing field. This means that if these women, women who are RNs, apply at these big companies, they are often welcomed with open arms.

Connect the Dots

Are you beginning to understand what I mean when I keep saying that there are numerous opportunities as a RN with the degree that you already have? To broaden your job horizons, you simply need to look at other employment venues than the traditional nursing employment venues. Look past the traditional nursing employment venues at a hospital, doctors office or clinic and nursing educational settings.

Okay. Back to Lopa. I bet you are wondering if it was a fluke, and it's just her college that is still teaching new grads to put clinicals on their resumes?

Oh, no. It's not.

Sadly, this outdated tactic is common everywhere.

Look at this before resume. With what you've already learned so far in this book, it may not surprise you to learn that nope, this new grad could not land a job either.

That is, not until he learned the current insights I teach on what to do with his resume, how to apply online, how to seek the opportunities that are all around him, how to use his resume to interview, and more.

Jay W. Gatsby
123 Main St., YourTown, CA 90210
(123) 456 7890
Jgatsby@gmail.com

Objective:
Seeking a challenging position as a staff nurse where I can contribute my strong leadership qualities, outstanding communication skills, and dedication to excellence attitude.

HIGHLIGHTS OF QUALIFICATIONS

- Superior performance award for the past four years in the Service.
- Trilingual-fluent in Ilocano, Tagalog, and English.
- Selfless volunteer-actively involves in the community.
- Adept at defining patient requirements and meeting their needs.
- Demonstrates competency as a care provider, communicator, advocate, collaborator, coordinator, manager, educator, and manager.
- Demonstrates pursuit and application of knowledge, respect for diversity, application of principles of critical thinking and scientific reasoning and informed moral and ethical decision making.
- Functions in professional nursing roles as a member of interdisciplinary teams.

OTHER EMPLOYMENT EXPERIENCE

ABC Military Base Clinic, YourTown, CA. August 2006 – March 2010 (40 hrs/wk).

Health Services Manager Key Duties

- Assisted in communication among beneficiaries, Primary Care team, network providers, and healthcare workers.
- Maintained 12,200 health records-created medical record, filed critical documents, copied records.
- Used AHLTA/Composite Health Care System to schedule appointments and maintained 9 provider schedules.
- Served as front desk customer service representative. Ensured patients needed were promptly identified and met.

- Establish work schedules and assignments for staff, according to workload, space and equipment availability.

CLINICAL EXPERIENCE

- Orthopedics Unit- ABC Medical Center, YourTown CA
  Jan2011-May 2011
- Pediatrics- ABC Medical Center, YourTown CA
  Aug 2011-Dec 2011
- Postpartum/Labor and Delivery- ABC Medical Center
  Aug 2011-Dec 2011
- Medical Surgical Unit-ABC Hospital, YourTown CA
  Jan 2012-May 2012
- Psychiatric- ABC Hospital, YourTown CA
  Jan 2012-Feb 2012
- Psychiatric- ABC Medical Center, YourTown CA
  Feb 2012-May 2012
- Community- 3HC, YourTown CA
  Aug 2012-Oct 2012
- Cardiac Unit – ABC Memorial Hospital, YourTown CA
  Oct 2012 – Dec 2012

LEADERSHIP

- President of the Volleyball Group. Effort leads to improve physical health of 94 members and created a positive environment around the town.
- Set the standard for excellence; Mentored and motivated 5 medical staff. All of them are soaring high and three were recipients of Air Force "superior performer."
- Led 3 members in identifying and shipping 1,078 records. Efforts led to the elimination of the backlog and gained 88 cubic ft in record's room space.
- Imparted vital computer skills through creating Composite Health Care System continuity binder for 9 staff-efforts led to increased clinic efficiency by 78%.
- Facilitated more than 182 hours for the running clinic-5 Airman improved their running times by 1.7 minutes.
- Augmented Warrior Health Flight by verifying and updating the health data records of 369 war fighters – efforts bolstered the 4th Fighter Wing deployment readiness.

- Led and organized bi-weekly fitness session for 92 personnel – contributed to 94% unit pass rate.

CERTIFICATIONS

- Cardio Pulmonary Resuscitation and Self Aid Buddy Care certified. Exp 05/12/14
- Advance Cardiac Life Support exp 03/23/15
- HIPAA
- Multicultural Awareness certified

ACHIEVEMENTS

- Fall 2012 Excellent Student Award
- Fall 2011 Excellent Student Award
- Military Achievement Medal 2010
- 5th Medical Operations 2009 Military Honor of The Year
- 5th Medical Operations 2009 Military Person of The Quarter
- 5th Fighter Wing Jul-Sep 2009 Volunteer of The Quarter
- USA 2009 Outstanding Achievement Award
- 5h Medical Group " 2009 Excellent Customer Service Award"
- 5th Medical Group Health Services Airman of the Month- January 2009
- 5th Medical Group "2009 Commitment to Excellence Award"
- Nominated for 2009 Military Health Services Manager of The Year
- 5th Medical Group "2007 Commitment to Excellence Award"
- Nominated for 2007 Military Health Services Manager of the Year

EDUCATION

- B.S. Degree in Nursing – ABC University, AnyTown CA Dec 2012
- A.S. Degree in Health Services Management – Community College of the Military Aug 2007

Results

You can see Jay's personal video testimonial at http://www.youtube.com/watch?v=5lcW4QOLzj8. Listen to him personally attest to the impact of a big bucks resume after months of no responses when he had been using the outdated techniques he was originally taught.

Cluttered Resumes

I have found the problem of cluttered resumes popping up all over the country.

Look at the layout in the example above and how challenging it is for someone to read this and the other "before" samples of new grad resumes that have been included in this book.

More than likely, these cluttered "before" resumes I've shown you are quite similar to your own resume, which could very well be filled with information that will hurt your chances at landing the jobs you're applying for.

Why?

Because the information you've chosen to put on your resume and the way you're showcasing it is not helping in any way to make you stand out.

Is your resume cluttered? Use the skills I've taught you here. Pull out your resume and go through the ingredient list. Find what mistakes you're making.

And then clean them up, one by one.

Your resume needs to showcase you, the candidate, as highly desirable or memorable. Let's take a closer look at how to accomplish this.

Pop Culture

Believe it or not, the key to making yourself desirable to prospective employers can be found in pop culture. Need proof?

Let's look at one of the biggest TV pop culture phenomena of all time: *American Idol*.

When Simon Cowell was on *American Idol* a few years back, one of his common critiques as a judge of the singers he heard was that they'd given a great performance, but they were not memorable. He said he would likely forget them.

The truth hurts, doesn't it? But the same thing is true in healthcare. If you don't find a way to make yourself stand out from the crowd, to make the recruiter who picks your resume out of a stack of dozens, or even hundreds, sit up and take notice of you, you're letting opportunity after opportunity pass you by.

The outdated resume techniques we've dissected so far are not helping these candidates to be memorable. The recruiter will not remember them because they are failing to stand out.

Sadly, I bet the same is true of your resume.

So how can you fix that? How do you make your resume stand out?

Skillset Transfer

The way to distinguish yourself on paper from the other resumes in the same stack as yours is to put the focus on your skillset. What skillset do you have? And not just in nursing, but from any line of work you have experience in?

If you can appropriately showcase the experience you have by transferring your skillset to the position that you are seeking in healthcare, you can land the nursing job you want. The trick is being able to highlight and showcase your existing skillset so that it mirrors the skillset that is needed for the job you're applying for.

We've touched on this a little in earlier chapters, but it bears repeating here. If you previously worked at McDonlad's, Macy's, or even The Body Shop, you have a skillset that hospitals and healthcare employers want: customer service.

Need a little help translating and transferring that skillset into the business of healthcare?

Let me show you how I would showcase such useful and important experience.

The Body Shop – Your City, IL **11/2011-01/2013**

Sales Associate

- Effectively interfaced with clientele and staff while successfully exceeding corporate sales expectations and interacting in a fast-paced and demanding environment at a top performing regional area store.
- Delivered high levels of customer service to ensure satisfaction and implemented successful problem-solving skills that surpass the expectations of modern day consumers.
- Consistently exceeded target sales goals by over 50% by developing solid partnerships with all levels of staff and clients.

If you really look at the words I've picked to describe the experience listed above, they are true of working both in retail and in a hospital. Both settings are fast-paced. Both have high turnover and are stressful. Both focus heavily on customer service.

Do you see now how you can take your experience from any work background and transfer your skillset to mirror what the healthcare sector is seeking in potential employees?

If so, welcome to knowing how to make the business of healthcare work for you!

This is how you will get you noticed, and yes, this will additionally make you memorable. And wouldn't Simon be proud of you!?!

Interviewing Off Your Resume

Not only will a big bucks resume get you job interviews, it will also help you succeed in those interviews!

A big bucks resume is individualized. And that is how a resume should be.

Having a cookie-cutter resume pulled from an online site or from a book will not help you in your interview, because the generic information from a cookie-cutter template doesn't highlight your specific skillset—your selling points that you'll use when answering the interviewer's questions.

True, anyone can write a resume. But having a resume written from someone with a nursing background infused with the business of healthcare is totally different. It is current. It stands out.

I know that much of what I have shown you goes against the grain from what you have heard about how to apply for nursing jobs, even at the school, college, or university you paid (or are still paying!) tens of thousands of dollars a year to attend.

But as we've learned, healthcare is changing in this country. And so too must the resumes of healthcare workers.

In this chapter, I have shown you how newly graduated RNs can make their resumes stand out and be noticed amongst a sea of applicants.

A bit later on, I will address the resume concerns specific to experienced RNs. But first, let me address something that all RNs need to know.

What is better left unsaid on your resume?

CHAPTER 5: How to Write a Big Bucks New Grad Nurse Resume

You have probably heard the saying, “If you cannot say anything nice, don’t say anything at all.”

On a resume, it isn’t that you are saying something that’s not nice. Rather, it is that you are not current with your insights on what not to say!

I want to pause here and point out once more, just in case you did not catch it in the “Acknowledgments” section, that the resumes used as samples in this book are real-life examples from real-life RNs. Again, I’ve simply changed their names and personal information to keep their identities private.

I want to bring this to the forefront of your mind so you can really begin to see what is actually going on out there in the marketplace, because it is sad.

In this chapter, we’ll focus on issues specific to writing a big bucks resume as a new grad RN.

Revamped?

Let’s look at another example—this time, a new grad RN’s “before” resume.

Diedra, the RN whose resume is next in our list of examples, had worked with me in the past. I actually spoke about her in my previous book, *Nurses, Jobs and Money: A Guide To Advancing Your Nursing Career and Salary,* when I explained how to gain experience via an internship that you can create for yourself.

Diedra had already graduated as a RN, BSN and was working. A young recruiter reached out to her, asking her to revamp her resume.

The following resume is what he put together for her.

DIEDRA O. WHY, RN, BSN
123 MAIN STREET
ANYTOWN, IL 90210
(815) 735-1766
WHY@YAHOO.COM

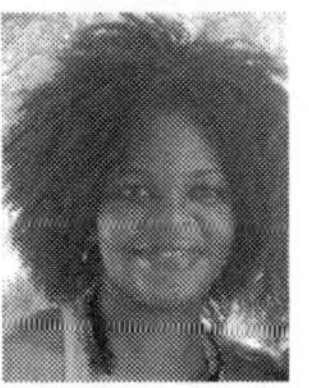

OBJECTIVE

To reduce my current work load of 80+ hours a week between two employers and become part of a dynamic healthcare team in a reputable organization where hard work & sincerity are appreciated and rewarded. Areas of interest include Home health, A&E, Cardiology, Critical Care, Gastroenterology, Nephrology, Neurology, General Surgery and Orthopedics.

EXPERIENCE

ABC HOME HEALTH Services, Any Town, IL - September 2013 to present
RN, Case Coordinator (full-time day shift)
Responsible for providing nursing care to ABC Home Health patients in a four county area. Travel an average of 600 miles a week to visit patients in their homes and provide medical services to a group of patients suffering from a wide variety of medical issues from surgical recovery to multiple sclerosis.

ABC CARE CENTER, Any Town, IL – July 2013 to present
RN (part-time night shift)
Organize and prioritize the care of 37 or more patients within a mixed rehabilitation, dementia and long term care setting.

ABC Inc- Any Town, IL – October 2005 to August 2008
SYSTEM SUPPORT SPECIALIST/ASSEMBLER (full-time)
Worked safely on a fast paced assembly line: 30-part assembly requiring organization, accuracy and efficiency. Charged with training new employees in a multi-tasked, detail-oriented and highly stressful environment focusing on standardized outcomes of production.

CREDENTIALS

- ✓ **ANY UNIVERSITY** – Any Town, IL - May 2013
  Bachelor of Science in Nursing
- ✓ **STATE OF ILLINOIS** – July 2013
  Registered Nurse

PERSONAL

Christian U.S. Citizen who is healthy, driven, hard working, honest, compassionate, caring, loyal, drug free and dedicated to my profession.

AVAILABLE UPON REQUEST

Supporting documents, credentials and additional background details.

Diedra laughed so hard at seeing what a staff nursing recruiter put together for her that she sent me this "revamped" resume so I could take a look and have a laugh too.

I was so glad that she knew not to implement the "insights" of this recruiter.

What's Wrong Here?

Oh my. There are so many things to choose from.

Let's start up at the top.

First off, no, you should not put your picture on your resume! And if you were to do this, it certainly should not be one that is a casual headshot with someone standing next to you and cropped out of view, with that person's hair still showing in the picture!

Although not needed, a picture on a resume should be a professional headshot. Period. Nothing else!

Let's reflect back on the ingredient list of a big bucks resume:

- Format and layout
- Name and initials
- Contact info
- Summary
- Experience
- Education

This will be a quick review as you are now learning what to look for.

Overall, the format of the recruiter's revamp is not bad, but I would recommend that the dates are put in the XX/XXXX format and moved to the far right.

Remember, for the name and initials, skip the middle initial. Bonus points for having RN, BSN!

Regarding the contact info, her address needs to be minimized so that visually, the most important contact information—e-mail and phone number—will pop out at the reader.

Per our understanding of the ingredient list, "summary" should be used not an "objective."

Remember, the potential employer knows that your "objective" is to land the job that you are applying for, so I would write a strong summary statement about your attributes as they apply to this potential future employer instead of an objective statement.

Your experience needs to showcase your impact at your previous employer. Again, this is a skillset transfer, but not a transfer of skills. It is imperative not to look average. Three bullets is ideal, but two to four is fine too.

Her objective statement is bad on so many levels—not only because it should be a summary statement rather than an objective statement, but because a far greater sin has been committed here. Let me show you why what was written here is so wrong.

No, I would not write about how you want to work less. Could you sound like more of a slacker? Yikes!

Remember, no one is going to read or remember 100 percent of your resume. So I certainly would not advise risking that the only part that gets read and remembered is that line about wanting to work less!

Yes, I agree that an eighty plus hour workweek is crazy, but to put this on your resume makes it sound like you are complaining and you are a slacker. Seriously, what if they did not bother to read the rest of the sentence?

Wow.

Next up, no, you don't need to put what shift you worked, let alone if it was part-time or full-time. The point of a resume is that you worked at a certain place for a specific duration of time.

Period.

Describe what you did at each place and add in the business of healthcare to showcase your results.

Think about it. There are nurses who show up, do their job, and that is about it. And then there are nurses who show up, do their job, and go above and beyond.

If you go above and beyond, you don't want to be lumped in with all the rest. Now is your time to highlight what you do and how well you have done it.

The result statements in the Experience section are the "how well you have done it" part. They are vital!

Education is on the ingredient list for a big bucks resume, not credentials. Again, skip the dates, and instead of highlighting your school, college, or university, make the reader visually notice the degree you have earned.

When you earned your degree is not important. What is important is that you have it.

Do you ever ask your physician what year he or she graduated from school, or ask where they went to school? Probably not!

Take the graduation year off of your resume. It won't help you, and due to the reality of age discrimination, it might actually hurt you.

Next we have "Personal" information. Really? This is 2014. Do I even need to address this? "Personal" information has no place on a resume. Get rid of it altogether!

When it comes to references, it is a given that you will supply them when and if they are asked for. Your resume is valuable real estate, and you simply don't have room to waste this, so skip that bit altogether. Get rid of them too!

What would I add?

Any of your EMR experience! I would showcase EMR experience as "nursing informatics." It does not matter if you are not a master at a system. Instead, what matters is that you have some insight into a particular system.

Overall, from this example, you can see what a young staff nurse recruiter told a nurse, and how I differ greatly in my recommendations.

So which one of us is right?

Keep in mind that if you are not a nurse and, what's more, not a nurse with business insights, you simply will not end up with the type of resume that will open the numerous doors of opportunity that lie outside of traditional employment venues for nurses.

This recruiter clearly sees RNs in only one type of employment venue: the traditional employment role of a staff nursing position. Again, there is nothing wrong with that if that is what you are seeking. But if you want to go for other positions in nursing, writing a big bucks resume is imperative.

Cover Letter Insights

If your summary is well written, you can literally copy the summary and use that as your cover letter. That said, if you can skip a cover letter, I would.

Why?

Because you want the reader to spend his or her time reading your resume, not skimming over the cover letter and tossing your resume aside.

Think about what behavior you are seeking—in this case, you want your resume read. From there, provide the appropriate amount of material to achieve the behavior you want to encourage.

If you want an employer to read your resume, then only give them your resume.

If you sort of, kind of hope they will read your resume, then provide them a cover letter as well.

If you absolutely must provide a cover letter, make the information the same or extremely similar to what is on your resume, so when the recipient is done reading the cover letter, they will realize it is the same or similar information on your resume at first glance, and they will start reading your resume farther down.

Genius!

As a nurse, you know you would not give a pediatric patient a full plate of food with the dessert on the same plate—not if you really wanted the protein and veggies to be consumed first. Why then would you give a ton of information all at once to future employers?

The pediatric patient asked for dessert, right? But did you give it to him or her right away? Of course not. The same idea applies here.

You need to learn how to overcome online job application hurdles by knowing what you really do and do not need to give hiring managers—just as you learned as a nurse what you really needed to do or not do depending on the outcome you seek to achieve.

Ulterior Motives

Diedra is a newer nurse, with not even one year of nursing experience under her belt, but she certainly would not go places with the resume this recruiter wrote for her.

I must honestly question if the recruiter wrote her resume this poorly so that the outcome would be that Diedra taints her marketplace with it and cannot find work. Then she'd have to go through the recruiter to find work.

Another possibility is that the recruiter is seeing garbage resumes like this one flooding the market for nurses, and he thinks what he put together will actually help Diedra, since it looks like all the other nursing resumes out there.

We've already covered why this is a poorly chosen strategy. The idea is to stand out, not to look average.

Or perhaps it is because this recruiter only sees nurses working in traditional employment venues that he wrote a resume for Diedra that was tailored to only get her noticed for these kinds of roles.

I'm not sure. I never spoke with the recruiter; I simply laughed with Diedra about the multitude of issues apparent on this resume and explained to her, as I have to you, why to never use these techniques in 2014 and beyond.

One last point. I don't want to hear that the faculty at your school or an HR person you know said your resume is good.

Again, really look at who is telling you that. What types of nursing positions have they done or assisted with? And what nursing resumes are they comparing yours to?

How much do they really know about the business of healthcare, and nursing in particular?

Go For Great

When it comes to creating a resume that will open the doors of opportunity for your nursing career, you don't just want "good." You want "great."

You don't want the same old options anymore, do you?

As I've said, healthcare is changing and so too should the resumes of healthcare workers.

It is time to step it up. Get your game on and be current!

This will get you the results you're looking for.

My Version

You may wonder, when it comes to a summary statement, what would I write?

I would go with something strong and businesslike:

Multilingual, determined, and results-driven experienced healthcare worker with solid and proven customer service skills engrained from previous work experience within a Fortune 500 company.

Documented team leader, self-starter, and problem solver with exceptional communication skills.

For both healthcare and non-healthcare work experience, I would incorporate the business of healthcare as I've shown you how to do.

ABC HEALTH – Any Town, IL **3/2012 to 7/2012**
Certified Nursing Assistant:
Routinely exceeded corporate expectations in patient care at the largest Catholic healthcare system in Illinois.

- Provided exceptional care to over 22 patients on a single shift.
- Management routinely entrusted my care of patients to meet and exceed workload of 25%+ while maintaining patient satisfaction and safety at or above corporate expectations.
- Daily interaction with successful inclusive and collaborative communication amongst a diverse socioeconomic and cultural clientele.

ABC, Inc. – Any Town, IL **10/2005 to 8/2008**
System Support Specialist and Assembler

- Key system support specialist within one of America's largest companies, a top 100 ranking company of the Fortune 500 companies, interacting exceedingly well within a corporate culture with high standards.
- Ensured availability of products needed to complete daily tasks.
- Charged with training over 10 new employees in a multi-tasked, detail-oriented, and highly stressful environment, while particularly focusing on standardized outcomes of perfection.
- Worked safely on a fast-paced assembly line: 30-part assembly (organized, accurate, efficient).

You Get What You Give

If you are not getting the results from employers that you wish for, it's time to reflect back on what you have been giving them and really assess the situation.

You need to speak to the business of healthcare in your resume, because as healthcare is changing in this country, the resumes of the healthcare workers must reflect this.

Formulate strong, results-oriented, business of healthcare statements that will yield dramatically different results from employers in your market when you write your experience statements.

In the next chapter, I will share an example of more experienced nurses' resumes. We're talking now about nurses who want to advance their careers in nursing, not just take an old school, lateral move in nursing to another, similar job.

CHAPTER 6: How to Write a Big Bucks Experienced Nurse Resume

The Carol Burnett Show, Donny & Marie Show, Happy Days, The Brady Bunch. No matter your age, you have probably heard of these classic TV shows.

Some things that are old become classics. And some things change.

Think about *Saturday Night Live*. It is very different now then it was in the past. Why? It needed to transform as time passed to grab the attention of the current audience.

The same thing applies to your nursing resume.

If you really want something different in your nursing career, your nursing resume needs to be different today than it was in the past. If you want the attention of different employers, if you want a career in nursing and not only a nursing job, the outdated way of writing a resume isn't going to cut it anymore.

You need a big bucks resume. In this chapter, we'll apply the principles of big bucks resume-building to the resumes of experienced nurses.

Classic

If you are happy being a classic, traditional nurse, then you should continue doing what you are doing—but beware. Even in the classic, traditional employment venues for nurses, the business savvy executives who now orchestrate those employment venues are looking at classic, traditional RNs in a different light.

Classic, traditional RNs are usually higher paid. And classic, traditional RNs who are higher paid are on thin ice in today's times. Why would I say such a thing? Because it is true.

The classic, traditional, highly paid RN, although he or she has fantastic experience to draw from, simply costs the business' bottom line too much money.

Reality Wake-up Call

If you are a classic, traditional RN, you may need a reality wake up call.

One in three hospitals across the US markets are slated to close in the next few years.

A quick Google search will show that this is already happening. My goodness, just Google "Hospitals closing in Hawaii" or in Long Island. If isolated island markets are losing hospitals, can you imagine what will happen in your local market?

I lived in Chattanooga, Tennessee for two years. There are

three hospitals in that market and only two hundred and fifty thousand people. With the Baby Boomers retiring and therefore jumping onto Medicare, the government healthcare payor, the government is becoming the biggest payer of medical costs—and all this before we factor in Medicaid and Affordable Care Act clients—and therefore, the government is cutting reimbursement rates to contain costs. Think about it. Of the three hospitals in a small market as Chattanooga, Tennessee, one of these hospitals is highly likely to close due to lack of funding.

I now live in Cincinnati, Ohio. There are numerous hospitals throughout the Cincinnati marketplace. When the news broke at the end of September 2014 that Southwest Regional Medical Center, formerly Brown County Hospital, in Georgetown, Ohio, sixty minutes outside of downtown Cincinnati, Ohio, closed its doors one week after pressure was placed on the hospital to pay its creditors, I was not surprised in the least.

But why?

How is this really happening?

Hospitals are taking in less than what they are billing.

The biggest expense for a hospital is the nursing staff. Again, it's just a matter of connecting the dots.

If the hospital can downsize their highest paid RNs, you bet they will. It is business. Plain and simple.

No, you do not need to agree with this practice. But you

do need to realize what is happening around you so you can be prepared to deal with it.

My first book, *Nurses, Jobs and Money — A Guide to Advancing Your Nursing Career and Salary,* addressed the closings of hospitals seen nationally. Do note, that book was published in 2012. In Georgia alone, the headlines in early 2014 showcased four hospitals that closed. Can you imagine what will happen as this trend continues?

So classic, traditional RNs, get ready—because your "stable job" is realistically not that stable. The good news here is that you have time to prepare for this upcoming problem, so I highly suggest that you do so.

That said, you cannot continue to just do the same thing in nursing anymore, because the landscape of nursing and healthcare is changing. That means it is time for you to change too.

Downsizing Experienced RNs

Take a look at this classic, traditional RN's resume. She is from New York, and like many across the country, she is faced with being downsized. This RN reached out to me, wondering what else she can do in nursing.

Although this is not spoken of often, the downsizing of experienced nurses is happening all over the nation.

Experienced, classic, traditional nurses simply cost too much money for the healthcare organizations they work for. To cut these high costs, the business savvy people who run these organizations are downsizing the higher paid nurses right and left.

If you continue to listen to the outdated advice and job-hunting techniques that are prevalent in nursing, you may find yourself unemployed.

Do I Need More Degrees to Be Marketable?

For most RNs, if they go through getting downsized, their response is to falsely believe that they need more and more pieces of paper—higher degrees—to be marketable. That too is an outdated notion.

Take a close look at this RN's resume and, based on what you've learned so far, see if you can spot the issues I found here.

ANDREA LOOKED OVER

PO Box 123 Any Town, NY 90210 * (123)456-7890 *
ANDREALOOKEDOVER@YAHOO.COM

Experience: Registered Nurse

ABC Hospital, AnyTown NY 90210 4/2012-current

- Vascular access team
- Placing Intravenous catheters in patients
- Care of PICC lines and all CVAD's within the hospital including dressing changes and trouble shooting
- Care and management of infiltrations and phlebitis as needed

ABC medical urgent care, AnyTown, NY 90210 12/09-current

- Charge Nurse in a busy urgent care
- All aspects of patient care adult and pediatrics

- Directing flow of patients throughout their visit including assessment and triage of all patients

ABC Medical University, AnyTown, NY 5/1998-7/2009

- Staff nurse on a medical surgical floor, including shift coordinator
- Emergency room PSL adult and pediatrics
- Preceptor to various staff and students
- Assist with various staff mandatory education
- CPR instructor within the hospital
- Assist as needed with hazmat training in the E.D. and hospital wide

Registered Nurse

ABC Health and Rehabilitation Center, AnyTown, NY 8/2000-4/2006

- Team leader on 40 bed acute rehab unit or 60 bed skilled nursing floor
- Charge nurse on 40 bed acute rehab unit or 60 bed skilled nursing floor
- Supervise building of 160 bed rehab/skilled nursing facility

Registered Nurse

ABC Healthcare agency, AnyTown, NY 9/2005-3/2006

- Staff nurse on cardiac critical care floor per diem at ABC Hospital
- Float to ICU at ABC Hospital

Education: ` **Bachelor of Science in Nursing,** December 2010
ABC Medical University, AnyTown, NY

Associate of Applied Science in Nursing, December 1998
ABC Community College, AnyTown, NY

Professional Certification: MyState RN license, CEN, CPR

References: Available at request

Sadly, the "before" resume shown above more than likely looks like yours.

It is outdated.

It is not truly showcasing what you do and the impact you make.

It is not standing out, and as a result, you will more than likely not be noticed or invited to seize the opportunities that are all around you.

To keep it visually similar, I put the "after" version of this resume in the same format I used for the previous "after"' resume I showed you—Lopa's resume.

Please understand, you can use just about any format you like. The important thing is to use a strategic and eye-catching visual layout and business-savvy wording. Your resume does not have to be in the format I am using here again as an example.

Please also note that this "after" resume is still partially incomplete, as more information was needed from this RN to fully implement the big bucks resume strategy here.

ANDREA LOOKED OVER

RN, BSN

YOUR TOWN, NY 90210
PHONE 123-456-7890 • E-MAIL
ALOOKEDOVER@GMAIL.COM

SUMMARY

Experienced BSN-RN. Responsible, experienced, enthusiastic, compassionate, and dedicated healthcare professional with a strong background of customer service, critical thinking skills and hospital experience seeking enhanced career opportunities.

EDUCATION AND LICENSURE

ABC Medical University – NY
Bachelor of Science in Nursing

Licensure – **Registered Nurse, State of NY**

EXPERIENCE

ABC Hospital – AnyTown, NY **04/2012 - Present**

Registered Nurse

- Successful utilization of critical thinking skills in organizing and prioritizing the care of 4+ or more patients in high acuity Medical-Surgical and ER nursing units

ABC Medical Urgent Care – AnyTown, NY **12/2009 – Present**

Charge Nurse

- Versatile and integral team member accepting a multi-faceted mix of healthcare challenged clientele
- Independent self-starter delivering exceptional patient-centered care in close collaboration with all the members of the multi-disciplinary healthcare team

ABC Medical University – AnyTown, NY **05/1998 – 07/2009**

Charge Nurse

- Versatile and integral team member accepting a multi-faceted mix of healthcare challenged clientele

CERTIFICATIONS, SKILLS, AND MEMBERSHIPS

- **American Heart Association Healthcare Provider CPR - BLS**
- **ACLS**
- **PALS**

NURSING INFORMATICS

- **EPIC**
- **McKesson**

Your Thoughts?

Use what you've learned so far to spot what is now working better in the above "after" resume. Revisit our ingredient list.

What changes have been made to the formatting and layout?

What changes could still be made to improve this resume still one step further?

Think like an employer. What information would you want to see here? Use this as a learning opportunity.

Add in the Business of Healthcare

Now you need to add in the business of healthcare.

How?

The key pieces of information to include here are the statistical data of how you are helping to cut costs, the measurable outcome of your work and expertise, what the patient satisfaction level was, and so on.

You'd better believe that including these kinds of details will make a huge difference!

Good, but Not Great

Believe it or not, some people are at least a little ahead of the game. In the case of this next example, I finally received a resume from an experienced nurse that really was not a total train wreck.

However, it still needed some tweaking to really get her noticed.

Look closely at her resume and see if you can spot the issues I found.

123 MAIN STREET
MYTOWN, IOWA 90210

PHONE 123-456-7890
E-MAIL
KBORINGS@AOL.COM

KIMBERLY BORING SNOOZE

WORK EXPERIENCE

ABC Hospice

Director of Patient Care- Any Branch

September 2009-Present

- Supervision, education and directing patient care staff to ensure delivery of quality comfort care to patients and families
- Communication of patient needs to physicians, staff, family and caregivers
- Assuring documentation of care and interventions meet Medicare conditions of participation
- Maintaining budget and staffing while meeting needs of patients and staff
- Development of relationships with physicians, hospitals, long term care facilities and civic organizations to provide education regarding hospice services.

ABC Veterans of America

Associate Director of Medical Services

February 2009-August 2009

- Performed site visits to

Veterans Administration Hospitals with spinal cord injury programs to assure quality care

- Medical advocate for Veterans with spinal cord injury

ABC Health System:

Interim Director of Access Management

July 2008-February 2009

- Worked in cooperation with senior management to assure budget guidelines were met
- Restructured department through the use of LEAN Process Improvement to contain cost
- Worked cooperatively with internal and external customers, facilitating transfers for patients with complex needs lines using clinical, organizational and interpersonal skills
- Used an integrated approach toward patient outcomes, utilized standards, guidelines and pathways for care delivery
- Incorporated data and information to continuously improve care and practice to enhance outcomes

Administrative Director

May 2007 – July 2008

- Provided direction and guidance to others regarding practice, assisted with decision making and problem solving
- Provided resources and support to staff in the application of clinical practice and case management
- Utilized guidelines, standards and research to support care delivery with optimal patient outcomes
- Incorporated data and information to continually improve operations
- Influenced improvements in practice settings by maintaining current standards

ABC Medical

Trauma nurse

November 2001-May 2007

- Provided staff nurse support in busy emergency department experiencing critical staffing shortages across the country
- Assumed charge nurse responsibilities and performed department triage
- Maintained appropriate certifications and educational requirements to provide care in Level 1 Trauma Centers for both

adult and pediatric patients with wide ranging illnesses and injuries

ABC Medical Center

Emergency Department Staff Nurse

January 2000 – November 2002

- Provided direct patient care to various emergency department patients
- Assumed shift charge nurse responsibilities including staff support patient flow
- Maintained appropriate certifications and educational requirements to provide care in Level 1 Trauma Centers for both adult and pediatric patients with wide ranging illnesses and injuries

EDUCATION:

ABC College of Health Sciences AnyTown, Iowa

Associates Degree in Nursing

LICENSE:

Registered Nurse, State of Iowa # XXXXXX

CERTIFICATIONS:

BLS for Healthcare Providers

ACCOMPLISHMENT:

2004 Aureus Medical Employee of the Year
2007 ABC Health System Excellence in Nursing

AWARD:

2010 ABC Hospice Case Manager of the Year
2012 Servants Heart February and June

Number of Applicants

We'll get to what I found in the above example in a moment, but first let's pause for a moment and get real. In today's job market, for every one position, how many people do you think apply?

One? Ten? One hundred? More than that?

I do not have the statistical data on this one, but it's a safe bet that for any job you apply for, the number is at least ten. And often, it's much, much higher.

To stand out, your resume needs to immediately catch the attention of the person reading it.

Who, What, and When

Go back and really look at Kimberly's resume. The reader must read down quite a ways even to see that Kimberly is a nurse! Sadly, this is quite common.

Kimberly actually did a great job showing what she has done at her positions, but there are no proof statements that show her results. Remember, this is key!

Think about it. You can say you have done "x," "y," and "z" at a job, but what was the impact of that? This information needs to be on your resume, since that is what demonstrates to the person reading it that you understand the blending of nursing with the business of healthcare. And that's what they are looking for.

The next mistake I see above is that Kimberly is aging herself with her outdated e-mail address. As we've covered, many RNs also age themselves by putting the date they graduated from college on their resume. Be sure to avoid both of these errors.

Again, there is no reason to give the potential employer any reason to disqualify you. Since there is no reason to give them this kind of information, and doing so could actually hurt your chances, simply don't give it.

Your goal is to have your resume lead to an interview and then to interview off of your resume to land a job.

If you are now noticing the kinds of differences I've discussed in this section in the sample RN resumes, well done!

Testimonials

Perhaps you would like to personally hear from others I have helped with their resumes and nursing careers. If so, visit these links on YouTube or search for Carmen Kosicek on YouTube.

https://www.youtube.com/watch?v=foFsHt-4DXE

Emily V., RN, BSN

http://www.youtube.com/watch?v=VwJdGyYtGFA

Sandra K., MSN, RN, FNP-C

https://www.youtube.com/watch?v=Sjphbybb6sM&feature=youtu.be

Manraj M., RN, BSN

https://www.youtube.com/watch?v=PaGPNG5aOiQ

Vanessa V., RN, BSN

https://www.youtube.com/watch?v=V1Kg94B5IRw&feature=youtu.be

Randy R., RN, BSN

http://www.youtube.com/watch?v=czcFAv66bpg

Stacie W., RN, BSN

https://www.youtube.com/watch?v=jeNtlgJ3jrY

Melissa M., RN, BSN

https://www.youtube.com/watch?v=vTtngvLSHoo

Lopa P., RN, BSN

https://www.youtube.com/watch?v=14ab06EHLb0

Julie G., RN, BSN

So many more on at Carmen Kosicek on YouTube!

https://www.youtube.com/results?search_query=carmen+kosicek

Remember, healthcare is changing in this country, and that means the resumes of the healthcare workers must change too.

I hope you are really catching on now!

If, at this point, you still do not understand that you need to do things differently, we may need to next assess if you are insane.

Let's discuss this in the next chapter!

CHAPTER 7: Common Misconceptions: What It *Really* Takes to Spread Your Wings

It's time for another reality check. Are you insane?

> *"Insanity: Doing the same thing over and over again and expecting different results."*
> ***-Albert Einstein***

I regularly run into new grad RNs who cannot land a job in nursing. They are spraying their resume all over and praying that they will get an interview . . . but nothing is working. Many of them are even considering looking outside of the nursing profession to land a job.

In this chapter, we'll examine some of the outdated and wrong-headed ideas that persist about working as a nurse in today's economic environment and look at why it's important to find someone to guide you through the crazy landscape of bad advice about your nursing career.

Tainting the Market

Do you realize that if you mess around too long in your current marketplace with the wrong resume, that you will taint your market?

Here's the problem. If you don't know what you are doing and you are applying online—as many employers now require—then your data has been captured and when the system has said "no" to you, you're stuck.

How then, will you be noticed by that employer a few months down the line, once you have reached out for help and returned to your job hunt using innovative insights like the one laid out in this book?

You won't. Not if you over-flood your market.

On the other hand, if you seek advice from someone who knows how to strategically build your base of experience wider in the short-term, can you imagine how the hiring manager at the job you really want will look at you the next time you apply?

You bet! He or she will be anxiously awaiting your application!

Still, be careful. The more you taint or contaminate your marketplace with outdated, stereotypical techniques on your nursing resume, the fewer employment opportunities you will have once you go at this game the right way.

Insanely Experienced

I hear from experienced nurses all the time who, no matter how they try, cannot escape the type of nursing they are currently doing. Often, they are at the point of considering either leaving the nursing profession altogether or going back to school for a higher degree in nursing.

By now, you should have a pretty clear image in your mind as to why I believe that this type of thinking is insane.

Clearly Insane

If what you are doing is not working, why would you keep doing it and believe that you will get different results?

As we have established, that is insane.

Why would more degrees make you more marketable when you cannot find gainful employment with the degree you already have?

That too is insane.

It won't.

Why do RNs think they must leave nursing to escape the traditional employment venues of nursing?

This is not the case—as long as you're aware of all the opportunities open to you with your current level of experience and education.

Many of the nurses I meet want to do something different in nursing, yet they never are afforded the opportunity to do so. Think about how many RNs you hear say that they are leaving, and yet they never do.

What I also find across the nation is that RNs really don't know what else they can do in nursing with the degree that they already have.

Many RNs are not even looking and applying for positions in the nontraditional employment venues that they could be working in—because they are unaware that they exist.

Why is that?

Sadly, it is often because they are using outdated techniques on both their resumes and their job searches. What's worse, many of these job seekers tend to be close-minded enough not to look outside of the bounds of traditional employment venues for nurses.

Why would these nurses persist in the false belief that getting another piece of paper, another degree, would land them into a different position in nursing?

Often, it will not. We'll explore this outdated belief more in the next chapter, but for now, let's look at some related issues and misconceptions.

More and More, Less and Less

More and more degrees are often required by traditional nursing employment venues . . . and yet they will pay you less and less as time goes by.

If you look outside of the traditional nursing employment venues, beyond the hospitals, doctor's offices, clinics, and nursing education programs, you can do so much more with your RN experience and the degree you already have!

The Bachelor's Degree

Let's clear up a common misconception right now. If you already have a bachelor's degree—in anything—I do not necessarily believe that you need another bachelor's degree in nursing.

If you want to stay in the traditional nursing employment venues for nursing then yes, you will need a BSN. The traditional employment venues will push you to get a BSN even if you already have a bachelor's degree in something else.

So why would I say you don't need another bachelor's degree?

Have you ever seen a job application that asks how many bachelor's degrees you have?

No, you haven't. They simply ask what your highest degree is.

If you do not have a bachelor's degree in anything and you are more than just a few years away from retirement—not retirement age, but true retirement—then yes, I believe you should go for a BSN, a Bachelor of Science in Nursing degree.

But what about those who already have a bachelor's degree in something else?

Not a BSN

Look at the resume of an RN from Florida who reached out to me. She is an experienced RN with a Bachelor of Science degree, just not one in nursing.

She could not understand why she was not getting the attention of potential employers.

Now you understand how to showcase skillset transfer and the results you have accomplished at your position, and how to speak the language of the business of healthcare.

Look at her resume below. What do you see there that might explain why no one was reaching out to her?

Go over our big bucks resume ingredient list, and reflect on that list while analyzing this "before" resume example.

Oh My-Please, BS, RN
123 Main Street
Your Town, FL 90210
123-456-7890
omp7@gmail.com

SKILLS SUMMARY

Active Florida Registered Nurse licenses with over seven years experience working in the acute care setting, understanding the processes and workflow common in this environment; solid customer service background that includes excellent interpersonal skills and the ability to interact positively as part of a multi-disciplinary team. Possess strong critical thinking and decision making abilities; highly analytical. Competent in managing multiple priorities and meeting deadlines. Excellent written and verbal communications skills. Experience working with various computer applications within the acute care setting as well as the business sector. Comfortable working with the internet and technology. Looking for the opportunity to transition into Clinical Informatics.

QUALIFICATIONS

CUSTOMER SERVICE

Competent in communicating with internal and external customers whether in person or by telephone to establish rapport, provide assistance and recommend solutions. Accustom to responding and resolving customer concerns, providing win-win resolutions in response to client inquiries. Responsible for company-client follow-up and liaison which include timely reviews, proficient multi-tasking and meeting tight deadlines.

INTERPERSONAL SKILLS

Proven ability to interact on a positive note with people of different cultures and personality types. Multi-disciplinary team participation in the medical sector and business profession. Experience working with clients in healthcare settings, home settings, as well as within various types of business environment.

ORGANIZATIONAL SKILLS

Demonstrate time management in providing excellent care for multiple patients utilizing considerable nursing assessment and judgment while giving prescribed care. Extensive involvement in healthcare and the business industry collaborating with team players for positive outcome/productivity.

TEACHING

Experience in providing clients the necessary knowledge and information by utilizing varied and appropriate teaching methods to accommodate the different learning styles of the typical adult learner.

PROFESSIONAL EXPERIENCE

Registered Nurse -	**ABC Medical Center, Your Town, FL**
	March 2013 - present
	ABC Health System, Your Town, FL
	January 2008 – August 2012
	ABC Health System, Your Town, FL
	July 2006 – April 2008
Home Health Aide-	**ABC Home Health, Your Town, FL**
	February 2005 – July 2006
PCA/Nursing Assoc	**ABC Hospital, Your Town, FL**
	July 2005 – June 2006
Prod Coordinator/CSR-	**ABC Printing & Advertising, Your Town, FL**
	November 2002 – January 2004
Acct Executive/CSR-	**ABC Company, Your Town, FL**
	February 2000 – March 2002

EDUCATION

ABC University - Your Town, FL

- Associate of Science in Nursing (highest honors)

ABC University- Your Town, FL

- B Sc in Graphic Arts Technology (summa cum laude)

ABC College - Your Town, FL

- Associate of Arts in Business Administration

REFERENCES

Available upon request

What's Wrong?

If you noticed that this resume is not showcasing this RN's results, great job! You are really getting the hang of this.

In addition, her resume is too wordy. This overwritten resume is not helping her to make a potential employer want to reach out to her.

Sadly, many RNs, just as this one in Florida, are planning to return to college and they are taking on massive student loan debt for an MSN, or a Master of Science in Nursing degree.

Numerous RNs, nationwide, falsely believe that the only way to get into a different facet of nursing is to have a higher degree.

Again, this is an outdated belief.

After this Florida RN worked with me, she realized that she could do so much in nursing with the degree that she already had!

For the record, even ADNs—Associate Degree Nurses—can do a lot with the degree they already have! True, it can be more limiting, as many employers do want a bachelor's degree no matter what field the job is in, but again, that is not always the case.

At this point, you really see resumes differently now, even for experienced nurses. And it's a good thing that you are, because this skill is vital in today's changing healthcare industry.

Now, what about the outdated belief in the necessity of more degrees? I will address this topic head on in the next chapter.

CHAPTER 8: You Can Make Your Existing Degree Work for You!

If you've read my first book, *Nurses, Jobs and Money — A Guide to Advancing Your Nursing Career and Salary*, you may already know that a close friend of mine is world-renowned electric violinist, Emmy-winning composer, and international recording artist, Mark Wood. The original violinist of the Trans-Siberian Orchestra, Mark is widely acknowledged as the premier electric-rock violinist of his generation.

In my first book, I spoke about Mark and how he has inspired me in my nursing career.

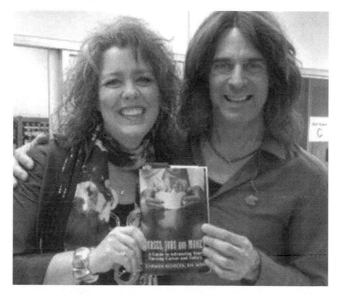

The reason that I bring Mark up again is so that you can realize it's okay to look at something as traditional as nursing—or in Mark's case, the violin—and to shake it up to where the traditional ways of doing things strategically fit into today's times.

Mark inspired me to disrupt the traditional market in nursing, just as he has done in the world of classical violin music.

A disruption literally uproots and challenges how we think, behave, do things, and how we learn about our day-to-day. In my case, that day-to-day is nursing employment.

In this chapter, I challenge you and other nursing professionals how they think about nursing education, nursing employment venues, job hunting techniques, online application strategies, interviewing skills, salary negotiations, and career advancement.

The education and experience you already have can take you further than you ever dreamed!

Rock It with What You Have

If you find yourself thinking of returning to school for a higher degree, I really want you to think twice about this and the reasons why you think it is needed to achieve your career goals.

No, I am not against higher education, but I am against getting a higher degree when you do not realize what you can truly do with the degree you already have.

I find it appalling that higher educational institutions will take money, including student loan money, from students of any age and not teach them how to showcase themselves appropriately to find employment with the degree they already have.

Look at this “before” resume from a fifty-seven year-old nurse in Mississippi.

OBJECTIVE:
A dedicated professional seeking a position as a Registered Nurse in a patient-focused healthcare environment.

PROFESSIONAL EXPERIENCE:

2013 **ABC Regional Medical Center**
Any Town, MS
Staff Nurse

- ICU/PCU RN

2010 **ABC Regional Medical Center**
Any Town, MS
Medical Technologist

- Generalist position responsible for testing in all areas of the laboratory

2008 – 2010 **ABC Medical Center**
Any Town, MS
Medical Technologist

- Generalist position responsible for testing and equipment maintenance
- Performed daily quality control in all areas of the laboratory

2000-2008 **ABC Trucks, Inc. / D & D Express**
Any Town, MS
General Manager

- Established primary in-house accounting system
- Managed USDOT compliance program

1995-1999 **ABC Regional Medical Center**
Any Town, MS
Interim Laboratory Manager

- Responsible for managing all clinical areas of laboratory

MT/QA Coordinator

- Managed all areas of laboratory quality assurance (QA)

1993-1995.01 **ABC Laboratory of America**
Any Town, MS
Laboratory Supervisor II - Hematology, Coagulation, Urinalysis, Special Chemistry, Serology, Bioveterinary Analysis

- Managed assigned sections of laboratory
- Assisted in the establishment of Bioveterinary Clinical Services for Southaven lab to consolidate veterinary testing and implement new assays
- Quality Assurance Committee member

Senior Laboratory Technologist II – Hematology, Coagulation, Urinalysis

- Performed laboratory analytical procedures as assigned by group leader

1992-1993 **ABC Community College**
Any Town, AR
Medical Laboratory Technology (MLT) Instructor

- Sophomore Level Course Instructor – Clinical Chemistry, Hematology, including practical labs and on-campus clinical rotation instruction.
- Team instructor in Fundamentals of Medical Laboratory Science, Selected Topics (sophomore), and Phlebotomy Certificate

EDUCATION:

Dec 2012 ABC State University
Any Town, MS 90210
Bachelor of Science in Nursing

May 2000 ABC State University
Any Town, MS 90210
Master of Business Administration

May 1983 ABC State University
Any Town, MS 90210
Bachelor of Science in Biology

LICENSES AND CERTIFICATIONS:

- Licensed Registered Nurse, Mississippi Board of Nursing, RXXXXXX
- American Heart Association Basic Life Support (BLS), 2/2013
- American Heart Association Pediatric Advanced Life Support (PALS), 1/2014
- American Heart Association Advanced Cardiovascular Life Support (ACLS), 3/2014
- American Society of Clinical Pathologist, Board of Registry, MT #XXXXXX, August 1984
- American Society of Clinical Pathologists, Board of Registry, MLT #XXXXX, August 1979

HONORS AND ACTIVITIES:

- American Nurses Association, Member XXXXXXXX
- Mississippi Nurses Association, Member XXXXX
- Sigma Theta Tau International, Pi Xi Chapter, ABC State University, Member
- ABC State University Robert E. Smith School of Nursing Student Nurses' Association (SNA), Member
- National Student Nurses' Association (NSNA), Member
- American Society of Clinical Pathologists, Associate Member
- ABC State University "Year of the Student", Volunteer

I wanted to scream from the mountaintops—and I could literally do that, since I lived in Chattanooga at the time—when I spoke to this nurse. We'll call her Janet.

Although she has an MBA and not one, but *two* bachelor's degrees, the reader has to dig way down to find this information in her resume. What's more, she was honestly considering going back to school to be an advanced practice nurse.

Janet did realize that, as of 2015, she would need a terminal degree—a DNP or PhD—in order to be an APRN. Janet also admitted that she currently has student loan debt and would have to take on even more to become an APRN.

Wow. I am continually amazed at the brilliant RNs out there who falsely believe that more and more pieces of paper will lead to more job opportunities. They will not.

After working with me, Janet learned how to showcase what she was truly doing at each of her positions.

She learned that she did not need any more education.

She learned how to search for nontraditional employment venues to utilize her existing RN and MBA.

Janet was incredibly excited after realizing the opportunities that were available to her in her current marketplace with the degrees she already had.

I have no doubt that, at this point, when you look at the "before" sample resume above, you can now see so many changes that you would make to this experienced nurse's resume to turn it into a big bucks resume.

A Sad State of Affairs

I find it sad that no one in the collegiate system had taught these skills to Janet—not during her studies for any of her three degrees. Instead, they taught her the false notion of needing more pieces of paper. This is simply no longer true.

During our conversation, I pointed out to Janet that the money—not to mention the time—it would take to return to school for another degree would be far better spent on funding her retirement. Janet whole-heartedly concurred.

Don't forget, employers are most often not offering pension plans in 2014 and beyond, so it is therefore up to the individual employee to save and fund his or her own retirement! If the return on investment of a new or different degree is not there, your money would be better off going towards your retirement. Period.

Applying Math

I am also in utter shock at the number of adults who do not understand elementary school math.

Numerous RNs reach out to me sadly, they are totally serious about taking on more student loan debt—Janet included.

It never occurred to these RNs that if they do not pay back their student loan debt—which often cannot be considered grounds for bankruptcy—that this debt will be taken out of future tax returns and even social security checks.

What's worse, if they default on their student loans, their RN license itself will be yanked, and they will not even be able to earn a living as an RN! Reread that...it is true. Any professional license, be it an RN, a real estate agent license, an insurance license, etc., can and will be revoked when the signer and/or co-signer of a student loan default on the payments!

The elementary school math looks like this. A BSN degree, if you are already an RN, runs an average of $5,000 - $15,000. An MSN degree generally runs an average $25,000 - $40,000. It should be noted that I am being quite conservative in these estimates.

The minimum student loan payments (before interest) for a seven-year payoff on a mere $10,000 worth of student loan debt averages out to $120 a month, Again, that is before interest for a BSN. For an MSN, with the average student loan debt of $30,000, that payment skyrockets to $350 a month before interest.

I have not even spoken of the terminal degree payments for a DNP (Doctorate in Nursing Practice) or a PhD. Those numbers are staggering! If you have amassed $70,000 in student loan debt, the seven-year note, before interest, is $830 a month!

Terminal Degree Recommendations

Those who continue to only look at the traditional routes of nursing often lean towards returning to school in order to become an advanced practice nurse. In 2015, the recommendation for this level of employment is a terminal degree: a DNP or a PhD. The nursing profession already realizes that this timeframe is unrealistic and the date has been extended past 2015, yet still, a terminal degree is the preference for APRNs.

I know. It is not required; it is a recommendation. But how is this recommendation going to affect someone who only has a BSN, who is thinking about long-term advancement in the field?

In many markets across the nation, the answer after looking at all those student loan payments is going to be thank you, but no thank you.

For the record, the American Nurses Association (ANA) is not grandfathering the diploma and associate's degree nurses in for the BSN recommendation by 2020.

So why would anyone believe that the ANA would grandfather in nurses with MSN degrees to the advanced practice nurse level to fit with that position's terminal degree recommendation by 2015 or whatever the target date is that they set? I don't believe they will.

Again, I am not against education. I am for education. But I am also all for showing RNs what they really can do in nursing with the degree that they already have.

The vast majority of the higher paid positions for RNs in nontraditional nursing employment venues require a bachelor's degree, but not necessarily one in nursing. There are even employment venues that do not require any degree, but simply the RN status.

If nurses continue to listen to the outdated beliefs that are still being taught to them—usually by nurses who have only pursued traditional nursing employment roles—then these nurses will continue to get more and more degrees without learning what they can really do in nursing with the degree they already have.

This saddens me.

Dare to Be Different

If you still want to go for more education, I really want you to think about something that—again—the schools do not normally speak about: where you will finish your degree.

Think about the wall of degrees in a doctor's office. More likely than not, those degrees are from different schools, colleges, and universities. Really think about that.

Why would they do that?

Getting the Best

As I've mentioned previously, I lived in Chattanooga, Tennessee for two years, previously I had lived in the Chicago-land market for thirty four years, the Detroit, Michigan market for seven years and now, I live in the Cincinnati, Ohio market. When I lived in Chattanooga, Tennessee, if I wanted state-of-the-art healthcare I would go to either Vanderbilt in Nashville, or Emory in Atlanta.

If a physician only trained at one of those places, I might view him or her as only having insights from one state-of-the-art medical facility. If, however, a doctor had spent time at both of those medical establishments for medical training, I would feel I have the best of both worlds in that physician.

Why then do nurses go to the same school for their BSN, their MSN *and* their PhD or DNP?

Honestly, I believe it is because no one has pointed this out to them, and the schools certainly won't do that, because they would stand to lose a lot of money if they did.

Think about it.

Foreign Nurses

What about the foreign nurses who come to the US?

This is interesting to me as well. I've helped several RNs who had a degree in nursing along with several years of nursing experience from their home country. Many of them have landed in the US and have passed the NCLEX. And yet they cannot land a job as an RN.

Often, these foreign nurses are encouraged by a school to get a BSN, perhaps fully repeating the studies they completed in their home countries. But is this really necessary?

This happens to physicians too. I know many physicians who are MDs in their home countries. They come to the US, do a fellowship, and pass their boards. Yes, this is a long process, but they are not expected to redo their entire education. And many of them go on to land jobs as physicians in the US.

So why is it different for the RNs?

It shouldn't be. Those who I've personally coached learn how to overcome this objection with potential employers head-on.

Stop, Look, and Listen

Stop listening to the outdated ideas being pushed by schools, colleges and universities. Instead, look at the real truth in the examples right in front of you.

Another common end-point considered by many RNs who do not want to return for more college education is to become legal nurse consultants or nurse entrepreneurs.

Again, I want RNs to really realize what else is out there. There is nothing wrong with being a legal nurse consultant, but LNCs need to massively market themselves. They also need ongoing continuing education to keep their certifications current. And yet this aspect of these jobs is rarely spoken of.

Again, this is the stereotypical route that nurses take because they do not realize how to transfer their skillset to the business of healthcare. This in turn opens up countless doors of opportunities for these nurses, using the degree they already have.

Yes, a nurse entrepreneur is a fabulous route to take, but again, I find that most RNs want a paycheck. They want to feel stable. If you know me, I am quick to point out that no job is truly stable.

That said, this desire for stability influences the kinds of jobs that most nurses are interested in. They want a position that makes them feel that there is stability for them in the form of a steady paycheck.

For more information and increased clarity on the many titles of nursing jobs and roles that I recommend considering, look at my first book, *Nurses, Jobs and Money — A Guide to Advancing Your Nursing Career and Salary*.

Additionally, you will find information there about how to search for those jobs. This second book was written to help you with the next step: arming yourself with the right resume to use to apply for and land those jobs.

Dare to Be Different

The need to stay current in today's marketplace makes it imperative to learn a different way forward. It is vitally important to learn from someone who has done what you want to do.

Likewise, it is important to learn from someone who has his or her finger on the pulse of today's economic environment in nursing—someone who knows what it takes to get you to where you want to be.

I've outlined why the outdated belief in the importance of more degrees does not necessarily solve the problem of finding gainful nursing employment in today's economic environment.

It should be crystal clear to you now that as healthcare is changing in this country, a new kind of resume is needed by job-seeking healthcare workers: a big bucks resume!

I've shown you how to take something as traditional and classical as nursing and put a current twist and flair into it. Now it is up to you to do so.

In the next chapter, I reach out to those who need help fully connecting the dots. Get ready to take these new insights and put them into practice to make a positive difference in your nursing career!

CHAPTER 9:
Keeping Nurses in Nursing

Chico's and Macy's are two of my favorite clothing stores. I know, most nurses would not shop here, because most nurses work in traditional nursing employment venues and need scrubs. But for those who seek a different path of nursing employment, they will usually end up shopping in stores like these.

One day, Beverly, a store clerk in the Chattanooga, Tennessee Chico's who had been helping me for a few seasons, asked what I did for a living. I told her I was a nursing career coach. She went on to ask more questions about what that specifically means, how I help RNs, and what has happened to those RNs who I've helped.

I explained further, and next Beverly asked me where I was ten years prior. You see, unbeknownst to me, Beverly was a nurse.

Ten years prior, she decided to walk away from nursing because she only knew about the traditional employment venues in nursing and she was tired—absolutely physically exhausted—from working in those venues. She did not want to go back to school, so she sincerely thought she was at the end of her nursing career.

Now, there is nothing wrong with being a store clerk—and I mean anywhere, let alone either of my two favorite clothing stores. And yet my heart was saddened.

All too often, I see nurses of various ages leaving nursing —either the new grad, who cannot find a job in nursing, or the experienced nurse, who does not know where else his or her nursing career could truly go.

In this chapter, we'll look at the reasons why many nurses—from new grads to experienced RNs—decide to leave nursing, the misconceptions that often lead them to do this, and how to broaden your own career horizons as an RN.

Stay in Nursing

It is my goal to keep nurses in nursing, be it at the bedside or beyond. America needs these nurses. There are so many roles that nurses can take to continue to impact patients' lives.

Again, sadly, these alternative paths are not openly spoken of by nurse educators and those who work in traditional nursing venues. Again, I firmly believe this is because the vast majority of nurses simply do not know about these alternative career paths.

This means that not only are they unable to benefit from such alternatives, but that they, in turn, as they progress to later stages in their careers and sometimes become nurse educators themselves, are unable to teach others about these exciting new opportunities—let alone knowing how to guide future nurses to learn how to land these positions.

Armed with my insights from this book and those I shared in *Nurses, Jobs and Money — A Guide to Advancing Your Nursing Career and Salary*, you should have a firm grasp on not only what roles are open to you as a nurse, but how to highlight your skillset on your resume in order to reach these positions.

As I continue to help more and more RNs across the country to take roles in the nontraditional nursing employment venues, I have no doubt that word will spread—not only through my work teaching other RNs, but thanks to those who I've helped, who will continue to go out and share what they've learned with others.

Yes, I do help nurses to find employment in the traditional roles and settings of nursing too, because many nurses are happy in those roles as well.

Even if you're one of these nurses, it's important to know and understand your options. You never know what the future holds.

Things Change

The hospital of today is not the same hospital it was five or ten years ago.

I look at employment roles in nursing quite differently than most. It is my goal to have more and more nurses realize the options that are available to them, rather than to see so many of them leave the nursing profession due to the mistaken perception that there is only "one way" to be a nurse.

My Wish for You

I sincerely wish for you to be happy in any facet of nursing you seek to work in.

We are not all cut from the same cloth, and therefore, we cannot all be expected to be happy doing the same type of nursing. And that is okay.

I wish for you to find your niche in nursing and make it your own.

I wish for you to spread the word to other nurses of any age or experience level that it is okay to spread their wings and fly, because the wide world of nursing is truly open to them.

I wish for you to help open-minded thinkers be heard in nursing, so that they will not be drowned out by those who cling to outdated thinking.

Nursing is a truly wonderful profession—especially when all the facets of nursing are revealed to us and we understand the different places our careers can take us.

I've said it before, and I'll say it again: healthcare is changing in this country, and so too must the resumes of healthcare workers! Change your resume today so that if and when you need it, you can apply with confidence and get yourself noticed for the position in nursing that will bring you true joy.

Learn More

> *"Finding a good mentor will help bring out the best in you when you don't necessarily see the qualities you possess. Talent cannot be taught which is why coaches are more valuable than players. Without good coaches, the importance of talent would be diminished."*
>
> ***--John Lang***

Carmen's vision is to continue to uplift nurses, as well as nursing students, to the complete spectrum that is obtainable within the realm of nursing.

Throughout this book, you have learned that the cookie-cutter format for a resume will not help you with your career in nursing —no matter who writes it for you.

A resume is only one facet of the overall nursing employment picture. For example, job searching, the game of online applications, interviewing, salary negotiations, and more all play a vital role in RNs landing the jobs they are seeking.

Remember, a resume needs to be personalized.

A resume is a working document for you to use—not just to get an interview, but actually *in* an interview—to strategically position yourself above the competition and help you land a job offer. You need to be able to interview off of your resume, using relevant examples of what you did and the impact you made doing it.

Your resume is simply not something that you can download from the internet. Nor can you simply pay someone to write it for you if that person never even speaks with you and doesn't understand the blend of nursing and the business of healthcare that is needed.

On the other hand, a resume that is personalized for you by someone with the insights needed to help you to get to where you want to go in nursing will take you far. You just need someone who understands what it takes to get there.

If you want a personalized resume from a nurse who knows how to take you where you want to be in nursing, be it in a traditional or nontraditional employment venue, reach out to Carmen at www.CarmenKosicek.com.

One of Carmen's Signature Program clients wrote:

Carmen,

My daughter's econ class has a program where they have to live "real" lives and survive on realistic salaries while paying realistic bills, mortgage and car payments etc.

The salaries for available jobs at the only factory in town were posted along with job descriptions and requirements.

She applied for "Shift Manager" due to her experience with leadership and other activities, along with eight other students.

Out of the eight, there were only three positions granted. Two students got Shift Manager positions (at $50,000/yr).

*My daugher got a new position that was **created because her resume was so fabulous** "Head Shift Manager" (at $55,000/year).*

Her resume was so amazing because I taught her how to use your resume writing techniques, skills, and tools to write it.

It took her FOREVER (probably six-eight hours total) to write, but it was worth it!

See the ripple effect here?

THANK YOU, Carmen!!!!
- Ann, RN, BSN in Spokane, Washington

The techniques that Carmen teaches are applicable in any career. As a nurse herself, Carmen reaches out to other nurses to teach them what they can do within the spectrum of nursing with the degree that they already have.

To work with Carmen one-on-one, or to contact her for career coaching on how to overcome the online job application, interviewing techniques, salary negotiations, and more, or for further information on how Carmen can personally help you with revamping your resume, go to www.CarmenKosicek.com.

Carmen welcomes groups of any size to invite her in for speaking engagements at colleges and other venues. Her talks and events are geared to show RNs how they can advance into higher paid and exciting new positions within nursing.

You can also join Carmen's professional network on NursesLounge.com and LinkedIn.com, or follow her on Facebook at https://www.facebook.com/NursingCareerProfessionals.

About the Author
Carmen Kosicek, RN, MSN

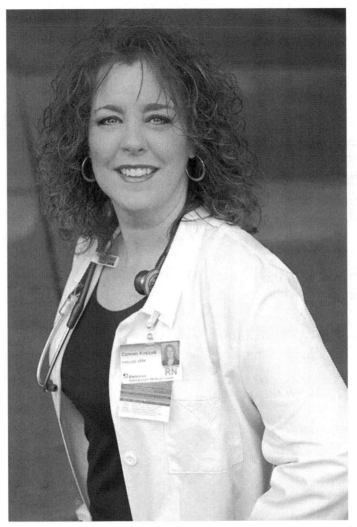

Carmen Kosicek, RN, MSN, has an extensive academic and professional background in the fields of nursing and healthcare.

Carmen has helped thousands of nurses and nursing students to envision a brighter nursing future filled with possibilities. With her love of business, she has assisted her nursing clients to increase their incomes by 20 percent or more within an average of five months.

Contemporary, passionate, and thought-provoking, Carmen challenges nurses with support, encouragement, and guidance to reach beyond their envisioned expectations. Using step-by-step techniques, she guides them on how they can position themselves in the nursing field for continued career growth and success.

Carmen explicitly presents a proactive, twenty-first century approach, affording nurses the opportunity to protect their coveted RN license within today's vicious litigious arena—above and beyond traditional malpractice coverage.

Educational Background

Carmen's career began when she earned an Associate of Applied Science degree in Nuclear Medicine from Triton College in River Grove, Illinois, a Bachelor of Science in Nursing from St. Joseph College of Nursing at the University of St. Francis in Joliet, Illinois, and a Master of Science in Nursing with a 4.0 GPA from the globally-recognized leader in nursing education, The Frances Payne Bolton School of Nursing at Case Western Reserve University in Cleveland, Ohio.

Carmen pursued her postgraduate education at one of the top fifteen Nurse-Midwifery and Nurse Practitioner programs in the country, Frontier University in Hyden, Kentucky, where she obtained a certificate as an Advanced Practice Nurse in Nurse-Midwifery.

Additional studies in healthcare economics and disease management led Carmen to a CMR certificate from the Certified Medical Representative Institute in Richmond, Virginia.

Intrigued by the expanding field of healthcare economics, Carmen studied under the Division of Insurance to expand her understanding of the insurance industry.

Healthcare Career

Carmen has also gained a wide array of practical, firsthand experience in nursing and business. Many of her inspirational insights come from the broad and strong knowledge base she built throughout her healthcare career.

Carmen started her healthcare career as a certified nuclear medicine technologist and went on to land her first BSN-RN position straight out of nursing school in women's health–labor and delivery in downtown Chicago, Illinois. She later became an OB nurse manager and finished her full-time clinical nursing career as an advanced practice nurse-midwife.

The business world pulled Carmen into healthcare sales. Eight years with Pfizer Inc., once the world's largest pharmaceutical company, gave Carmen solid, foundational knowledge of the field.

Keeping active in traditional nursing employment venues via Maxim Healthcare Services, the largest privately held healthcare staffing company in the nation, Carmen's healthcare experience expanded in the arenas of maximum security prison nursing, hospice nursing, and community health nursing.

Then collegiate education came calling. For eight years, Carmen taught nursing as a professor in both ADN and BSN programs in the private and for-profit sectors.

Carmen later became the Director of Nursing & Health Professions Program Research & Development for Corinthian Colleges Inc., one of the largest post-secondary for-profit education companies in North America.

With her solid and proven track record, Carmen went on to accept a position as one of only 120 national clinical nurse educators pediatric sales specialists on a contract for Johnson & Johnson/McNeil at a leading global provider of best-in-class clinical, commercial, and consulting services for pharmaceutical, biotech, and life science companies, inVentiv Health, Inc. After impacting the market one year longer then the original contracted timeframe, Carmen ranked 426% of goal.

Accepting the Associate Dean of Nursing in collegiate education, Carmen relocated to Ohio to further positively impact nursing.

Carmen is a contributing author for Publishing Concepts, Inc., the largest publisher of State Board of Nursing journals in the United States. Her articles and innovative insights span twenty-one states and, quarterly, reach a staggering 2.1 million nurses, students, faculty, and hospitals officials.

She is also a contributing author for the *Tennessee Nursing Extra*, the most respected and widely read healthcare journal in the state. There, her articles reach over one hundred and fifty thousand nurses, students, educators, and healthcare professionals of every degree and discipline across the state each quarter.

NursesLounge.com features Carmen as their sole and leading career coach. Join Carmen at NursesLounge.com today. It is a professional networking site exclusively focusing on nurses!

Carmen has been featured on NBC, ABC, CBS, and Fox News for her innovative career-coaching program that affords current market insights for RNs and step-by-step guidance from resume revamping, navigating the online job application, interviewing techniques, salary negotiations, and more!

Her first book, *Nurses, Jobs and Money — A Guide to Advancing Your Nursing Career and Salary,* is a must-read for every nurse and everyone who is one and/or wants to become one!

Carmen's second book, *Nurses, Jobs and Resumes – Resume Revisions for RNs From the New Grad RN to the Experienced RN,* directly incorporates how healthcare has changed and therefore how nurses must change her/his resume to keep pace by incorporating the fusion of the business with healthcare in today's economy for continued opportunities in nursing.

Nurses, Jobs and Money and *Nurses, Jobs and Resumes* are available on Amazon.com in print and e-book for download to computers (Windows PC or Mac), tablets (iPad or Android), smartphones (iPhone and iPod touch, Android, Windows Phone 7, BlackBerry), and Kindle devices.

Family

Carmen is a mother of two teenage children and a wife of twenty-four years and counting. She resides in Cincinnati, Ohio, and enjoys time with her family and rescued ex-racing Greyhound, Nikky.

Contact

For further information on how Carmen can personally help you with revamping your resume, go to

www.CarmenKosicek.com.

To work with Carmen one-on-one for career coaching on how to overcome the online job application, interviewing techniques, salary negotiations, and more, contact her at

www.CarmenKosicek.com.

Made in the USA
San Bernardino, CA
26 January 2016